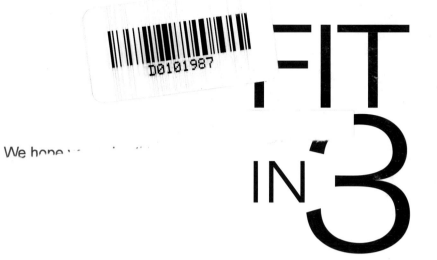

We hope

FIT IN 3

The Scandi Plan

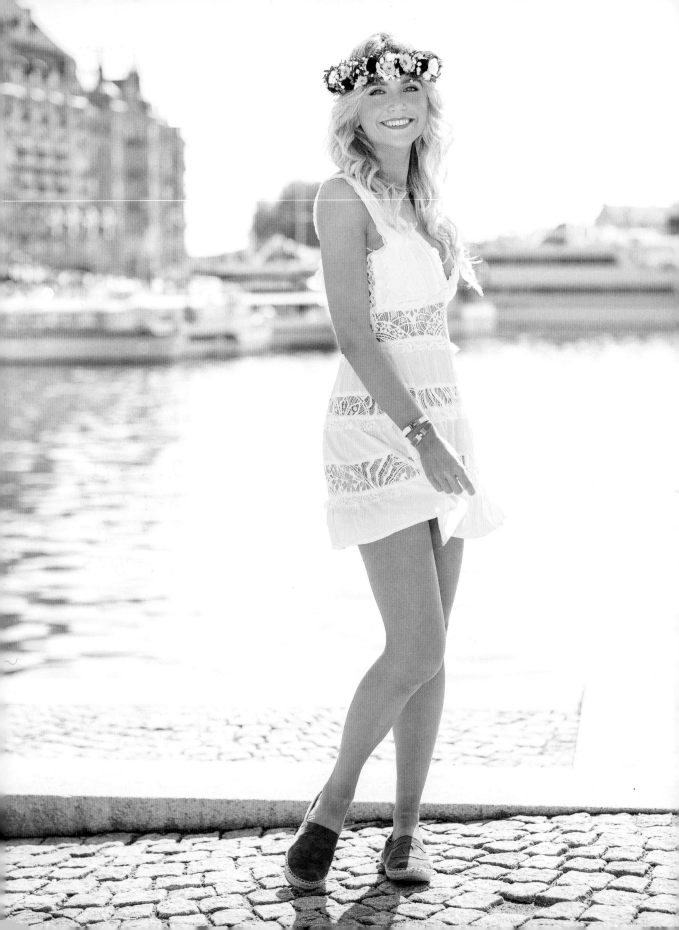

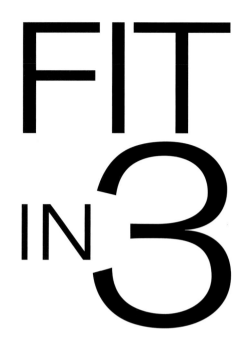

FIT IN 3

The Scandi Plan

HOW TO EAT WELL, TRAIN SMART AND ENJOY LIFE THE SWEDISH WAY

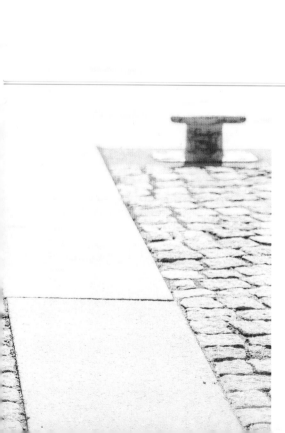

FAYA NILSSON

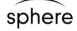

sphere

Fit in 3

First published in Great Britain in 2016 by Sphere

A CIP catalogue record for this book is available from the British
Library.

ISBN 978-0-7515-6677-2

Printed and bound in Germany by Mohn Media

10 9 8 7 6 5 4 3 2 1

Book creation and design by Harris + Wilson Ltd

Editorial Director (Sphere): Hannah Boursnell
Recipe Developer: Nicola Graimes
Food Photographer: Kate Berry
Consultant Nutritionist: Claire Baseley

Papers used by Sphere are from well-managed forests and
other responsible sources

MIX
Paper from
responsible sources
FSC® C104740

Sphere
An imprint of
Little, Brown Book Group, Carmelite House,
50 Victoria Embankment, London EC4Y 0DZ

An Hachette UK Company

www.hachette.co.uk

www.littlebrown.co.uk

NOTE: When using the recipes, use either metric or imperial
measurements, but not a mixture of both. Ingredients are
medium-sized unless otherwise stated. Every effort has been
made by the author to ensure that all the information in this
book is as precise and up-to-date as possible at the time of
publication. It is recommended that before changing their diet
or fitness regimes, readers always consult a qualified medical
specialist for individual advice and to ensure any conditions
specific to the reader are addressed. The author and publishers
cannot be held responsible for any errors and omissions that
may be found in the text, or for any actions that may be taken
by a reader or any injury or illness caused as a result of any
information contained in the text.

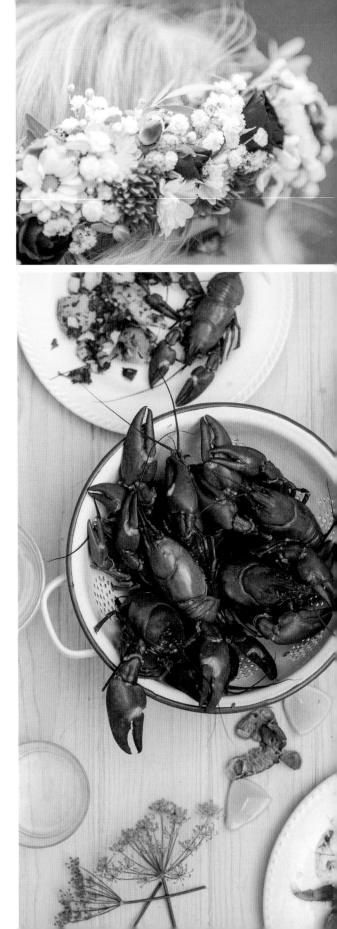

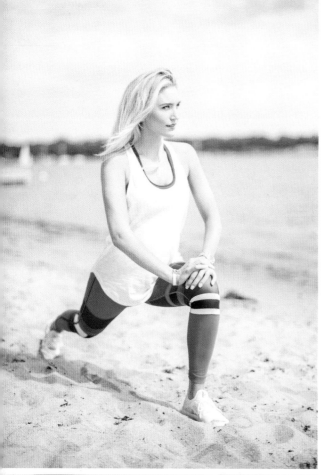

CONTENTS

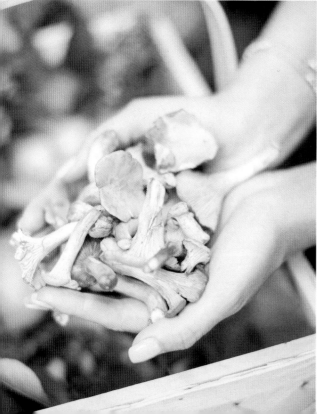

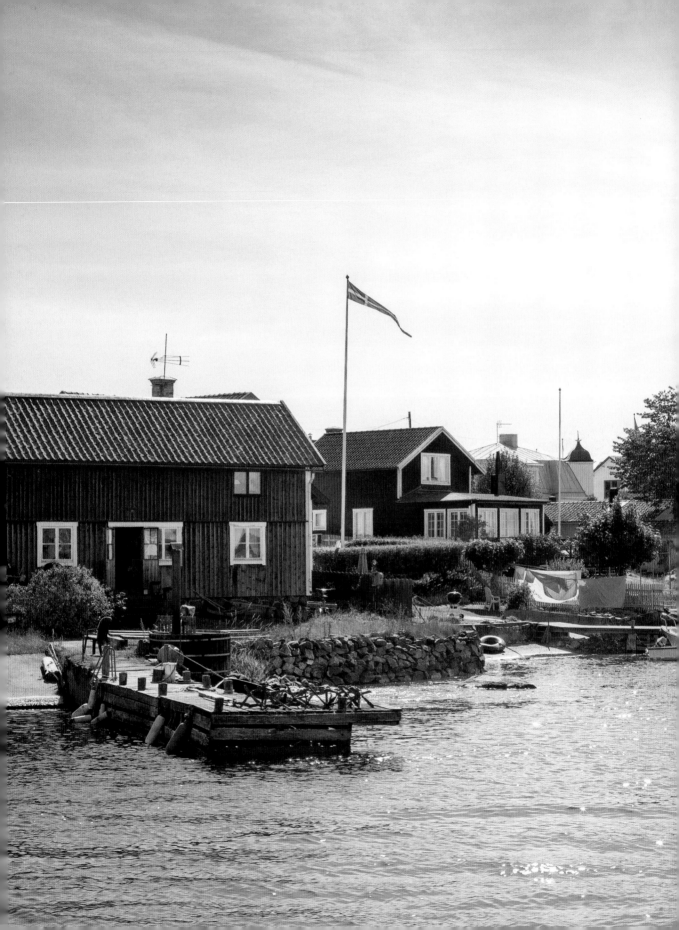

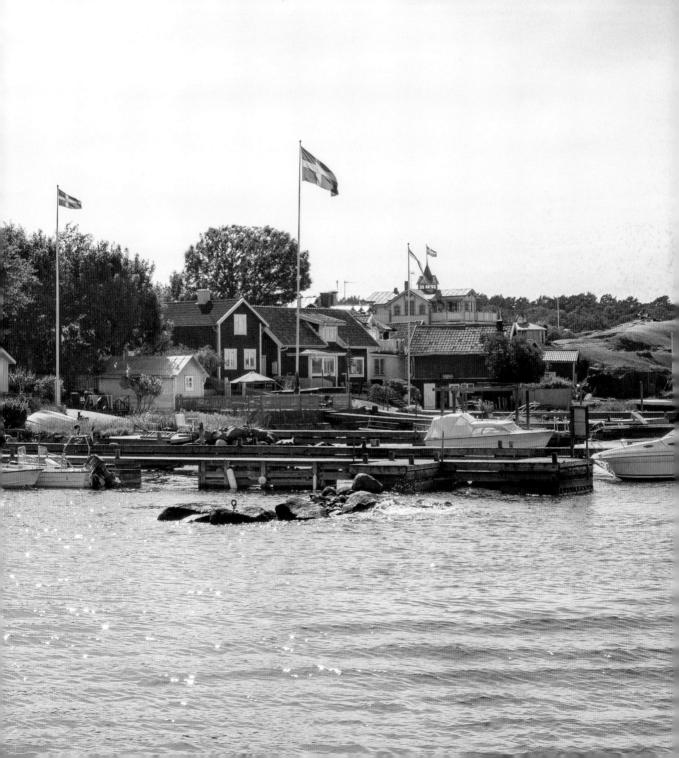

VÄLKOMMEN TILL SVERIGE!

WELCOME TO SWEDEN!

INTRODUCTION

When I was a small child growing up on a farm in the rural Swedish Arctic, I had sticks for toys and horses for company. Writing a blog or a book about a 'healthy lifestyle revolution' would have been as foreign to me as England was back then. But looking back on it now, my upbringing was all about health: fresh fish, fresh air, regular exercise and boundless nature were all part of my daily routine, as were the outrageously delicious cakes my mother used to make. Influenced by these pillars of Swedish culture (particularly the latter!), the blog I went on to start three years ago, *Fitness On Toast*, is a celebration of that holistic Scandinavian upbringing.

I've been working as a personal trainer in London's West End for over a decade now. When I started the blog, it was meant to be a part of this work – a place to share my wellness advice with clients outside of our limited hour together. But it quickly grew, developing a community of its own and taking me on some wild adventures. Over the years I've been lucky enough to meet many of the people who read *Fitness On Toast*, even trained with some of them, and made close friends as a result. I've travelled to many beautiful countries, interviewed people I idolise, and won some very flattering magazine awards. I now work with some of the world's top brands in fitness, fashion and travel, but through it all that Swedish kid's ethos remains: fresh fish, fresh air, regular exercise, boundless nature and outrageously delicious cakes…

I know what it takes to effect drastic and lasting change because I've seen it work for many in the past, myself included. I wavered at university – ate unhealthily, lazed about and forgot my heritage. This left me feeling sluggish, dissatisfied and lacking the motivation to live my life to the full. When I decided to make fitness my profession, I slowly unlocked the key components to a healthy and balanced life, using the positive habits of my childhood as a starting point. I'm really excited to share what I've learned with you here.

WHY *FIT IN 3*?

The first thing I've learned? Forget the tired notions of crash dieting and endless sit-ups – the world evolved beyond those a long time ago, *because they don't work*. As obesity and diabetes started becoming a bigger threat to public health, we were told that the solution was to cut out fats and spend every waking moment in the gym. But we now know much more about nutrition and fitness than ever before, and we've learned that there's a far more empowering approach, which will see you successfully live the healthiest version of your life. Contrary to the low-fat diet ethos (which almost always means 'high sugar'), fats can be good for you, and are in fact vital to living a healthy life. And short, smart exercise, coupled with the right mindset and good food choices, are much more effective than long hours on the treadmill. This book will show you how to combine these three aspects in a rewarding, sustainable and healthy way.

Consider, if you will, that there are two extremes to the theoretical 'spectrum of fitness'. On the left reside the Couch Potatoes, gorging on refined sugars, shovelling down simple carbs, and seldom exercising more than their remote control trigger-finger. On the right are the Fitness Fundamentalists, who drink protein shakes, eat six small pre-prepared meals a day, and are gym-bound for hours on end. This book will make you into neither of the above. I am no muscular hulk nor do I wish to become one, and likewise my blog's not exactly called *Fatness On Toast*. The ideal lifestyle is centre-right on this spectrum: toned, healthy, athletic, happy and balanced – able to enjoy life's delicious treats without falling down the rabbit hole, and adequately prepared to get back on track after an inevitable (even encouraged) setback. During my career as a personal trainer, I've seen and helped hundreds of clients, both male and female, make these discoveries and arm themselves with the right knowledge so that they can confidently achieve balance with minimum sacrifice. With *Fit in 3*, you can do this, too.

What's the big secret? I've deconstructed the complex formula into three simple components and *Fit in 3* will lead you through how to make the most out of each of them. Afterwards, you'll look back on choices you once made, and be thankful that you now make them differently, equipped with a new clarity of thought and better-informed understanding. This is the product of more than a decade's study of the fitness industry, all the professional wisdom I've assimilated, the handy tricks I've encountered, and all the hyper-commercialised myths I've unearthed as nonsensical – and believe me, the industry has plenty of those!

My simple formula looks like this:

MINDFULNESS + NUTRITION + EXERCISE =

SUSTAINABLE WELLNESS

It's as easy as 1, 2, 3. Allow me to elaborate…

THE POWER OF THREE

Three is the magic number. We're on the third rock from the sun; the moon has three phases, and the time and space we occupy has three dimensions. In sport, the three fastest win medals; there are three primary colours and three movements to a concerto. Artists and photographers compose the most beautiful images using the 'rule of thirds'. Architects design the strongest bridges from triangular frames. Convincing arguments are structured using three key points. Slogans lean heavily on this, too (think of the Olympic motto: *Faster, Higher, Stronger*), as does the ubiquitous three-letter acronym (BBC, JFK… OMG!).

The purpose of this little aside is to note the permanence and enduring nature of the triplet. It is a universal constant and, simply put, the brain finds three an easy number to digest. So, *Fit in 3* isn't an accident. This book is intentionally structured to highlight the holy trinity of a healthy life: **1** MINDFULNESS, **2** NUTRITION and **3** EXERCISE. Diving into *only one* of these three would be like trying to light a fire without kindling or oxygen! Pursuing all three is the key to sustainable success, and it's a really simple formula to apply.

In my experience, office workers will often train hard in the gym and try to eat right, but perhaps because of high stress levels and therefore lack of sleep, will struggle to reach their fitness goals. I often find that many aren't even aware that this is why they're being held back, and with a bit of guidance and a few tweaks, they can make progress quite readily. Equally, many former clients would train hard, but were drinking heavily and eating out in fancy restaurants, and/ or snacking on autopilot at the office, without considering their significant calorie surplus. And nowadays we have access to an abundance of fresh vegetables and exotic superfoods, but without the knowledge of how to best harness their nutrients, and the discipline to complement them with a regular and diverse training regime, the best intentions will fail. Awareness is a key weapon in the arsenal of the 'fit and healthy', and it is my hope that this book will arm you with that in spades.

To my mind, it honestly *can* be as easy as 1, 2, 3. Above all else, the key is to ensure you set yourself an easy path to follow, sprinkled with a little structure, dusted with a little planning and underscored with a little discipline. It then becomes an easier way to live, within the confines of gentle rules, rather than a scattered, last-minute approach that can see you floundering. You *will* feel better for it. Take 5 minutes out of your day for meditation. Go to bed an hour earlier. Drink an extra litre of water. Do some

regular, targetted exercise. The combination and application of the principles in this book will help you to become the healthiest version of you, for the long haul.

Yes, it may seem intuitive; cynics might even think, *We've heard that message for years!* Perhaps, but it's the *understanding* of each of these three elements that often gets lost in translation. Crucially, you need to know how to *apply* the learning to your everyday routine – not just this week or month, but for ever. This will unquestionably lead to an improved quality of life. It will give you more energy, a more resolute outlook, and will help you to face challenges, both physical and mental, in peak shape. This is where you start to train the mind to think in a new way, to approach your healthy choices from a logical and informed place, and then to form habits that genuinely stick. It's the best way to ensure a healthy life through youth, middle age, and retirement. Once you've understood and adopted these principles you'll find that you'll automatically lose that excess weight, tone up, and feel in tune with your body's needs.

You don't need to be fit already, you don't need to spend a fortune on this healthier life, you needn't be twenty-something years old, and (crucially) you don't need to give up chocolate! Anyone can participate, and this book will arm you with all the fundamental knowledge required to understand how to do it *for ever*. The results range from and include lean muscle gain, a reduced body-fat percentage, and a more harmonious sense of wellbeing. It's effective and incorporates workouts around your lifestyle, takes into account your time-poverty by being short and sharp, and helps you achieve the healthiest version of your life. Let's get started…

HOW TO USE THIS BOOK

Step 1 is complete: you now own the book! Step 2 should be the easier part: using it. The benefits it aims to deliver can be summed up as 'a kick-start to your healthier life, for the rest of your life' – so nothing too ambitious, then!

Fit in 3 contains three easily digestible chapters, plus a three-week daily plan to help you get started on your life-long journey.

1) MINDFULNESS, OR *REFRESHING THE MIND*

The mental approach is a hugely under-appreciated component of the healthy life. It's a way of thinking and understanding, informed by an educated appreciation of some home truths, and it governs everything else, including your training, your eating – and your willpower. We all waver, deviate from the course; that's to be encouraged, because it ultimately keeps us sane. To live a life of monk-like restraint is neither sustainable nor enjoyable; this section of *Fit in 3* will tackle, among other things, body confidence, meditation, sleep and yoga.

2) NUTRITION, OR *NOURISHING THE BODY*

I believe that healthy eating is and should be delicious, pleasurable, colourful and vibrant. When properly planned to include all the key nutrients, what we eat has a dramatic impact on how we look, feel and function. In this section there is a collection of easy-to-make, nutritionally balanced recipes for breakfasts, lunches, dinners, desserts, snacks and juices, using easily obtained,

fresh and cost-effective ingredients. By eating these nutritionally balanced meals, not only will you feel more energised, your skin will glow and you will naturally lose excess weight. To stay on track for life, you can't blindly restrict yourself – that's a direct course for failure – but you can't gorge daily either. This section will help you walk that tightrope: healthy snacking on the go, cold-press juices, why and when you should embrace fat and carbs (and which are the good fats and carbs to enjoy), how to sustainably enjoy sugar, why to drink more water, why to cook with spices (instead of sauces), why you should treat yourself regularly and how to read the food labels. It's preparedness 101.

3) EXERCISE, OR *TRAINING THE FRAME*

This section will introduce you to the reasons to train, the different types of training, and the benefits of doing so. Importantly, it'll look at how to keep things varied, because the best way to fight gym-fatigue is not to go there so often! Instead, the great outdoors can be a more engaging and equally gruelling workout; think hiking, sailing, skiing, running, power-walking, swimming and far more. It'll also introduce you to High-intensity Interval Training – *aka* HIIT – which will mean you never have to do more than 15 minutes of cardio again. Through a combination of diversity and intensity, along with perseverance at the start, you'll be able to comfortably work this into your routine.

Finally, there's my three-week training plan. You can do this from the comfort of your own home – no gym membership required! Creating lasting habits takes time, but you can do it more easily with informed decisions, a realistic approach and some good, old-fashioned consistency. The three-week training plan (in Chapter 4) is designed to help you get started, and it utilises your bodyweight to tone-up muscles. You might not quite have that six-pack by the end of the three weeks, but you'll have achieved something way more important – you'll have started your journey to life-long health, enjoyed yourself along the way, and those illustrious abs will come! Correct training is the priority, and that should be functional, safe and effective. My three-week plan debunks all the common misconceptions, most notably that 'healthiness' requires countless hours of mind-numbing cardio. Instead, we'll interweave the techniques you'll uncover throughout the book to create a healthy and sustainable lifestyle.

To ensure you get the most out of the plan, try to structure your week so that you make training a priority (as if it were a meeting) and so are less likely to cancel or miss a workout. For example, if you're doing low intensity on day three, why not get up a bit earlier than usual and walk to work to chalk up your fitness goal before the day really gets going?! On the rest day, try to do the Sun Salutation, which will ensure your body gets properly stretched out. If you'd like to give the plan a whirl, it also suggests a juice power-shot, a breakfast, a lunch, a snack and a dinner recipe for each day of the three weeks. You'll find all the recipes you need in Chapter 2.

In fact, you could use the book simply as a treasure trove of recipes, should you prefer. They are all delicious and nutritious Scandinavian-inspired dishes that have been developed alongside a professional nutritionist to ensure they're appropriately balanced.

Even if your interest lies in nutrition, hopefully you'll dip into the training section, too – and vice versa. You might want to use the book to re-educate yourself on the benefits of sleep, rest, recovery and other often neglected elements of a healthy and happy life. There's something here to pique any interest, and hopefully enough to keep you coming back to the book time and again.

For whatever purpose you use the book, I hope you love it!

Faya x

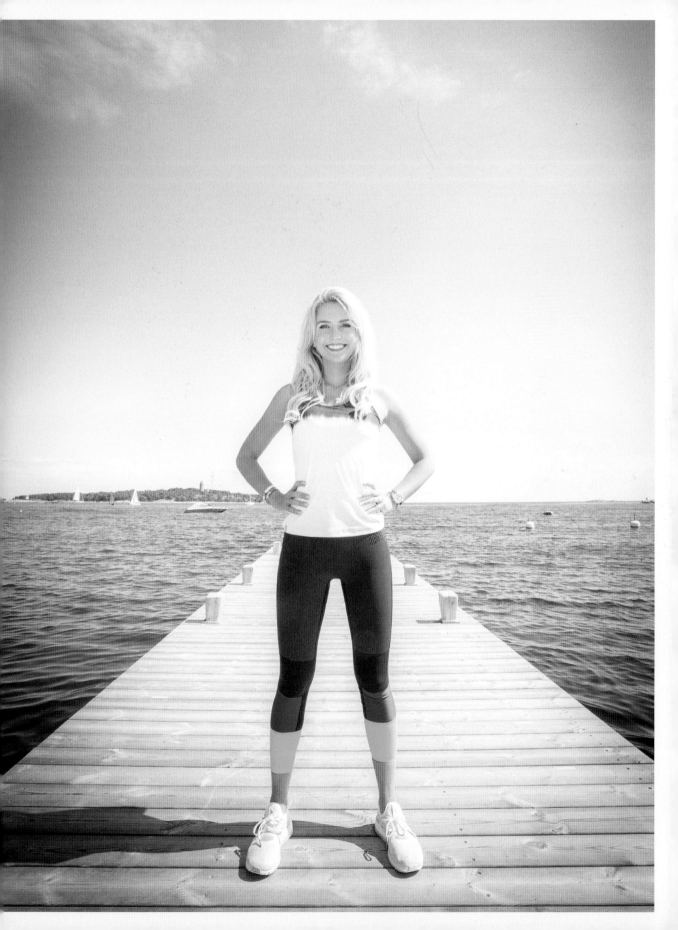

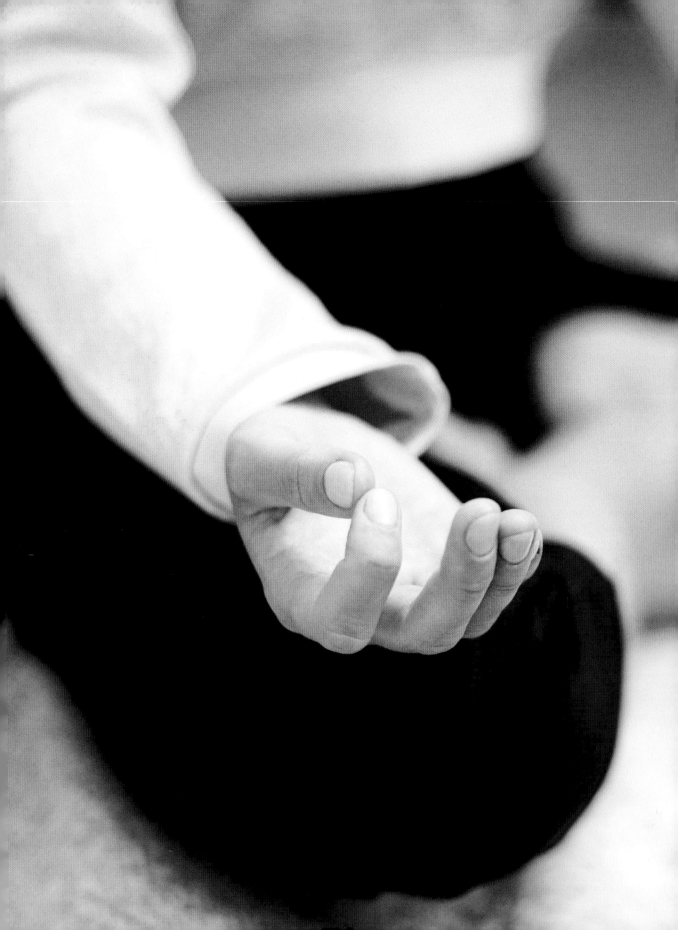

CHAPTER 1

Refreshing
THE Mind

'The very essence of mindfulness
is to observe objectively, to reflect
and to pay attention…'

WHAT DO WE MEAN BY MINDFULNESS?

What is mindfulness? Well, to manage your expectations, it has nothing to do with Jedi mind tricks – unfortunately, you won't develop superhuman powers of persuasion or learn to bend spoons! But, with a bit of practice, you will be better able to deal with the rapid pace of modern life and the overwhelming influx of stimuli that most of us now face on a daily basis.

MAKE TIME TO TRAIN

I believe that if we do something merely for the sake of doing it, we often risk doing more damage than good. Try to create the right amount of time to complete your training sessions safely. Seek to avoid rushing through your exercise in order to 'power out a cheeky shoulder routine', because you may tense the body, or suffer poor form and incorrect technique, which are likely to end up in injury. For me, it's far more about quality rather than quantity, and the focused thinking that comes from mindfulness totally complements this.

In one respect mindfulness might be seen as 'stepping back'; removing yourself from the hustle and bustle for a few moments every day, and concentrating on yourself. In fact, the very essence of mindfulness is to observe objectively, to reflect and to pay attention to both tiny details and your place in the bigger scheme of things. You are not disengaging from life, but rather re-engaging in a more conscious way, and living truly 'in the moment'.

If mindfulness techniques are woven into the everyday fabric of your life, they can bring a reduction in stress, a growth in compassion, a greater sense of calm and an appreciation of others and of the self.

HOW TO BE MINDFUL IN YOUR EVERYDAY LIFE

I believe there are four fronts on which we all can harness mindfulness to realise our aspirations for a healthy life: awareness, nutrition, fitness and breathing.

AWARENESS

Being able to recognise the nature of our thoughts is no easy thing. Emotion takes over and can obscure our ability to be objective. But the way that you think about your training and your healthy life can have a huge impact on the effectiveness of what you're able to achieve. It's fairly obvious that if you're really not geared up for your gym session and think you're going to have a lousy one, that'll probably come to pass — and vice versa. That begs the question, are you truly aware of what your attitude might be as you run into your session, and how it might affect the results? Research conducted in 2012 showed that twenty experienced runners exposed to positive feedback about their form, performance statistics and progress via headphones every few minutes were around 20 per cent more efficient in their consumption of oxygen by the end of the session, versus the control group. How can you replicate that in your own life? I find that meditation in the morning (a few moments spent in quiet contemplation) is a wonderful way to achieve insight into my own thought process, as it allows me a slice of dedicated time where I can just wander aimlessly within my own thoughts, testing some, being carried by others. Practising this in conjunction with breathing techniques, I always think my gym sessions are that much more effective!

NUTRITION

You've had a chaotic day at home with the kids and now you're eating the leftover fish fingers off their plates. Or maybe a stressful day at work has finished late again, so you've tried to pack in a 20-minute makeshift gym session and now you're racing to grab a sandwich, which you'll gobble down on the train home.

Take time to eat your food, not in front of a laptop or the television, but at a properly laid table. Set aside a dedicated chunk of time. (With the best will in the world, it may not be practical to do this every night, but even once or twice a week will make a difference.) As you eat, consciously appreciate the textures, flavours and scents in each mouthful. Perhaps think of it the way you would in a restaurant, where you might seek more 'value' from each mouthful. Try to savour and relish each individual piece of food, morsel by morsel, by consciously focusing on the diversity of flavours, the range of textures, the effects of temperature. Move the food about the plate to see how its form reacts. Focus on its aromas, the sounds it makes, how it looks…

FITNESS

Applying mindfulness to your fitness goals is all about making a connection with your body, seeking a form of body awareness. These days the most popular forms of training focus on efficiently blasting out as quick a workout as possible – including many of those in this book. High-intensity workouts very much have their place in a modern, busy life and I'm a big advocate of their benefits, but with more introspective and patient practices such as yoga, I get to access instant feedback on how my body is doing.

IMPROVING DIGESTION MINDFULLY

Focusing on the often overlooked details of your food heightens your sensory experience of your meal, but it also has far more practical consequences. A slower pace of eating improves the digestive process, as more salivary enzymes are produced in the mouth, helping to break down the food properly. Further still, it takes around 15 to 20 minutes for the brain to send the 'I'm full now' signal to the stomach – a slow and steady approach to eating means you're less likely to keep on gorging when really you're already full up! On top of that, stress can be a trigger for over-eating, so the pursuit of any practice that minimises stress helps with appetite regulation, too.

I've long thought that emotional stress can in turn affect the physical body, which creates more stress; a negative feedback loop, if you will. If the mind isn't aware that the body is stressed, how can it correct it? By being aware, you can help yourself to turn it into an advantage in any situation. Breathing is just something we do on autopilot, but focusing on it and relishing its restorative capability can make a huge difference.

Do I feel sore? Is there any tension in my shoulders? Am I overly stressed out? The body is very clever at highlighting imbalances as it's performing yoga poses. I would advocate trying to replicate this sense of connection in all your training. Think about exactly what muscle you're using and visualise where that is on the body – the diagram on page 143 can help with this. Can you contract the muscle and make the movement more efficient, more targetted? How does the rest of your body feel while you're moving in a certain way? Are you leaning on one hip or standing tall? By asking yourself these questions, listening to your body's answers, and maintaining this focus on mindfulness as it relates to your training, you'll help to increase the effectiveness of your workout.

BREATHING

When I'm stressed, I tend to hold the air high up in my lungs. My chest feels constricted, my whole body is set rigid, girded for something, and my breathing becomes shorter, sharper and shallower. That's totally normal, and if it rings a bell, then you're probably a human being. The first step towards combatting this is to stay mindful of your breathing and to recognise when those short breaths start, or you feel the rigidity set in your body; many of us have become conditioned to hold ourselves in this hardened manner. As soon as you recognise poor breathing technique, the ancient Chinese qigong method of deep and smooth breathing can prove extremely powerful. It advocates conjuring air from deep within the belly (which engages the large muscles in the diaphragm, massaging your internal organs and keeping them functioning nicely), inhaling through the nose and exhaling fully through the mouth, and is so effective that even in full-on fight-or-flight mode, you can totally relax your wound-up posture. It simply requires a mindful awareness of your chest, your muscular tension, your belly and your emotional state. Easier said than done perhaps, but chances are this happens more frequently than you might think, so I'd encourage regular breaks during which you close your eyes, sit comfortably and take a minute to breathe deeply and smoothly. I find that sitting cross-legged, fully upright, in a simple meditation pose or entering the Child Pose (see p.154) are incredibly conducive positions from which to breathe deeply.

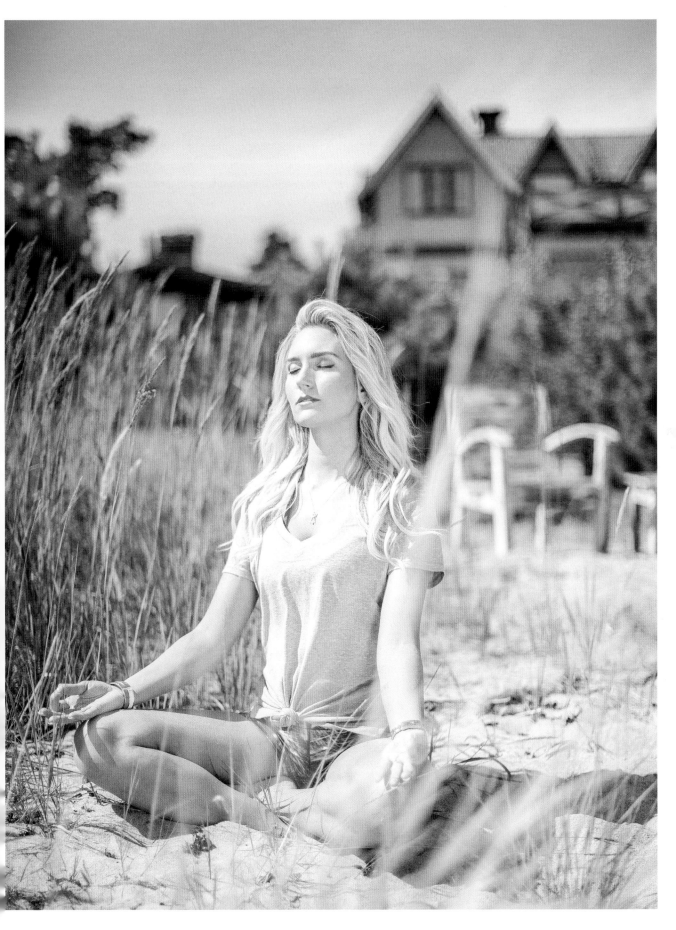

SLEEPING WELL

A good night's sleep is one of the most under-appreciated yet critical elements of a well-balanced, healthy life. It's the ultimate mental housekeeping operation, but many simply see it as a piggy bank into which they can dip when they need to borrow a few hours here and there. Studies have shown that a whopping 60 per cent of the UK population doesn't get enough sleep at night.

SLEEP CHEMISTRY

Our remarkable bodies operate on a circadian rhythm, which is finely tuned to the 24-hour cycle. As the day passes and our sleep debt grows, our minds are flanked by an ingenious two-pronged assault – on the one hand, a chemical called adenosine builds up in the brain during our hours of wakefulness and increasingly hinders our ability to function properly, forcing us to slow down as the day wears on. On the other hand, as darkness falls, the brain releases melatonin, which relaxes us and tells us to go to sleep. By the time we wake afresh the next morning, blood levels of these chemicals have fallen to their lowest, and the cycle begins again. We cannot escape this natural chemistry.

WHY SLEEP MATTERS

You might think that missing a few hours sleep is not a problem: I'll just sleep a bit more on the weekend. But you can't bank sleep and you can't recover what you've missed. The consequences of cumulative sleep debt are physical: your immune system weakens; you have diminished energy; your concentration wanes; your metabolism slows; you feel sluggish; you might want to eat more; you'll probably grow moodier and more stressed… and you'll almost certainly lack the motivation to train.

Scientists recommend on average eight hours sleep a night. My view is as follows: whatever amount enables you to feel wide awake and fully functional the next day is the right amount for you.

A TIME TO RECOVER AND REPAIR

When you train, you actually create microtears in your muscles. Afterwards, the muscle thinks 'Wow, that was pretty hardcore, I'd better strengthen up for next time!' Tissue renewal speeds up during sleep – after eight hours of slumber, your body is more than ready for tomorrow's training challenges!

WAYS TO SLEEP BETTER

Nothing guarantees a perfect night's sleep, but the following ten steps will certainly help to set you on the right track.

1 BE CAFFEINE SMART Try to avoid caffeine (from coffee, tea, fizzy drinks and so on) after 2pm, as it interferes with your natural neurochemical processes, including those that lead to sleep.

2 DOWN TOOLS The blue light emitted by phones and tablets interferes with the production of sleep hormones. Surrender your technology for at least an hour before you go to bed.

3 TRAIN EARLY While exercise releases a whole host of calming endorphins and promotes relaxation, working out late at night can disturb the quality of your sleep. Earlier is better.

4 EAT LIGHT A light meal before bed will create less digestive discomfort and shouldn't tax the natural processes too heavily while they're trying to operate on reduced-power mode.

5 BE NEITHER HOT NOR COLD The optimal temperature for good sleep is supposedly between 18 and 20°C (65–69°F). A window left slightly open and cotton nightwear and bedding can help regulate your nighttime temperature.

6 USE SCENT Anything that helps to promote calm and relaxation is generally something I like to work into my bedtime routine. I'll often dab a few drops of a sleep-friendly aromatherapy oil (such as lavender or chamomile) around my pillow.

7 WELCOME DARKNESS Darker is better! Light affects the quality of the sleep you're getting, never fully enabling you to enter the quasi-hibernating state of active sleep. Blackout blinds or a sleeping mask can help to kill pesky bedroom light pollution.

8 FIND THE RIGHT MATTRESS We spend over 35 per cent of our lives in bed, so it's worth investing in a comfortable mattress that will enable high-quality, uninterrupted sleep. It's an investment from which you benefit every single day (or night!).

9 BE MINDFUL If you're finding it difficult to fall asleep or you wake in the middle of the night and can't fall back asleep, use some deep mindful breathing to relax. Lying awake and worrying about your lack of shut-eye will make sleep even more elusive.

10 REPEAT Your body clock adapts to a regular routine, so going to bed at a similar time each night (with provision for the odd night out, of course) helps trigger sleep when you need it.

As we say in Sweden, *God natt*!

'Whatever amount of sleep enables you to feel wide awake and fully functional the next day is the right amount for you.'

EMBRACING BODY CONFIDENCE

There isn't a person on this planet who doesn't want to change *something* about the way they look – myself included. In a society in which unrealistic and sometimes unhealthy body ideals – in advertising, on social media, in movies – have led to intensified 'self-measurement', it's totally normal to feel insecure about your body. Recognising that we that *all* share these worries is the first step towards embracing a more confident outlook about what you *do* like in yourself. Here are some additional tips to help you combat those 'body-doubt' demons.

'COMPARISON IS THE THIEF OF JOY'

It's so hard not to compare yourself to others, but I firmly believe there is no 'ideal' body. So instead of focusing on others, shift the focus from how your body looks to what it can actually *do*. Can you play with your kids without struggling for breath? Can you lift a heavy box without asking for help? Can you get up from the floor without groaning? Who cares if your legs are a little short, or your hips a little wide, if you're strong and healthy? Despite all our negative thoughts about our bodies, they work super-hard for us. A healthy body is something to be truly thankful for.

HAVE FUN! BE POSITIVE!

As children all we cared about was how fast we could run and how high we could jump. We exercised without knowing that's what we were doing and without self-consciousness. Bring back the fun in movement and aim for that simple joy again! I find that, generally speaking, men are better at this than women. A man might say, 'Awesome work! I ran hard, sweated and smashed it.' A woman might say, 'I still have so far to go.' For me, it's all about seeking out the enjoyment in the training you do; focusing on the positives. Visualising yourself as strong and confident, standing tall and powerful with a smile on your face will help make that your reality.

BE KIND TO YOURSELF

Too often we talk about how dissatisfied we are with our own bodies. Thinking it to yourself is like self-torture and saying it out loud is like underlining it with a black marker pen. Think about how you respond when a friend voices her body insecurities aloud. You build her up, encourage her to focus on what makes her beautiful and unique. Be that good friend to yourself – don't allow the bully in your mind to have the last laugh.

BE THE HEALTHIEST VERSION OF YOU

Your health and fitness are things you can control and rely on throughout life, and are completely independent from anything and anyone else. You know your body better than anyone else, and only you can say when you feel strong, awake, alive and happy. My advice, for what it's worth, is to find the place inside you that joyfully celebrates your freedom. Don't let anyone tell you they think they know better, don't try to conform; just be the healthiest version of you!

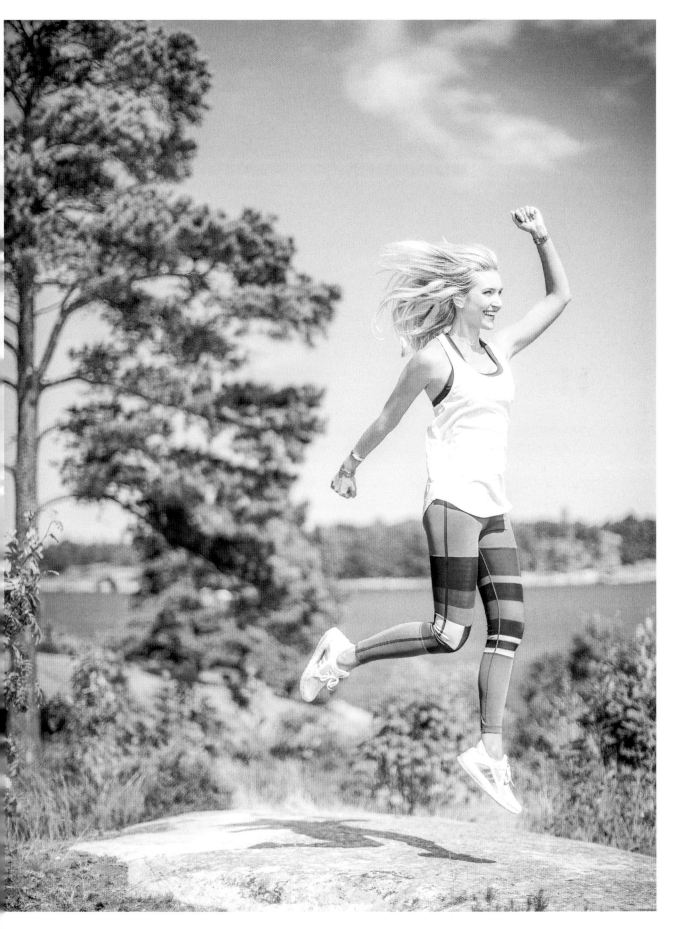

ACTIVE AND PASSIVE MINDFULNESS

Active and passive: both are states of 'mindfulness' and are essentially the same at their heart, but with subtle and incredibly helpful differences. Their similarities are to encourage a connection with the moment (an appreciation of the now) and to promote a 'watching introspection'; they're both peaceful pursuits. What's more, you don't need to check into a retreat in Bali to achieve these states of mind. They're also grounded in scientific study and are a serious form of mental practice.

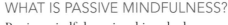

WHAT IS PASSIVE MINDFULNESS?

Passive mindfulness is achieved when you simply allow yourself to drift on the gentle ocean currents of your thoughts, not paying too much attention to what it is you're considering or where you're going; you're just floating in whichever direction your mind takes you, and it feels tranquil, weightless, serene. This is what most people classically consider to be 'mindfulness', and it's wonderfully impactful as the brain can be put into autopilot 'response' mode. It requires a degree of alertness to external stimuli, be they birdsong, wafts of air, your breaths, or vibrations or scents. But it also requires the ability not to become too involved in any one stimulus, to allow the mind supple flexibility to keep roaming freely, to skim about. Every time you start to consider something in too much detail, the mind must glide onwards to the next gentle impression, before swaying onwards again. Successfully practising passive mindfulness is a masterful exercise in observing rather than restricting thought.

DRAWING AND DOODLING

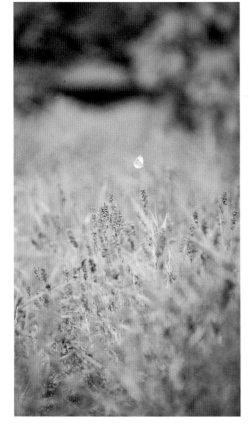

As a child I would spend hours on end sitting in the garden or forest with my watercolours. I was at peace with myself and the world around me. Some of my happiest, most contented moments have been spent all by myself, with my imagination for company. As children, we're captivated by the world around us, and inspiration flows freely through our veins. We're not afraid of making mistakes and therefore we happily explore, and let our creativity flourish. As we grow older, the fear of making mistakes and of being judged causes doubt and self-criticism to enter our minds; we're educated out of our youthful creativity. Drawing books for adults have become some of the fastest-growing and best-selling categories in today's bookstores. Adults love to doodle,

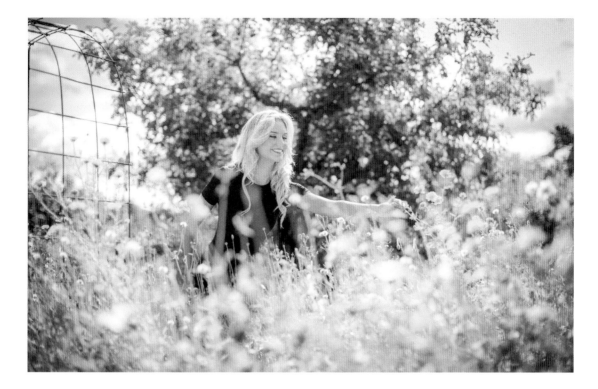

proving perhaps that creativity has not fully left us, but is simply dormant; we can re-learn it, rediscover it and we still have that youthful urge to explore. In a world that is so results-orientated, where mistakes are 'bad', colouring, drawing and doodling have become what many describe as therapeutic activities, providing time to completely drift away, relax the mind and just be present in that moment, bouncing from impulse to impulse. Drawing, unlike doodling, requires more intent concentration – perhaps allowing the mind to drift even further. To this day drawing remains one of my favourite ways to practise passive mindfulness.

WHAT IS ACTIVE MINDFULNESS?

Active mindfulness is much more about conscious observation; the higher reasoning in the mind recognising behaviours, stimuli and experiences that may trigger an emotional response, and working to dissolve them before they have a chance to grow. It's a practice of paying attention, and focusing the mind so that it identifies potentially adverse situations then neutralises them. Active mindfulness is a key component in many stress-relief practices. You notice, and then adjust in order to keep the mind focused on a single, balanced point. This is zoning in, whereas passive mindfulness is more about fading out. By means of more structured activities such as dance, cleaning your apartment, breathing, yoga and running, you are able to detach and witness, while also being engaged in activity.

YOGA

Yoga is the ultimate in active mindfulness, because it asks you to be a 'mental witness' while you're physically active; the mind is laser focused, and the body is in the moment. The Sun Salutation, over the following pages, works the entire body, while also focusing the mind. I've included it in the book not only so that you can dip into the multiple benefits of yoga, but also because even doing 5 to 10 minutes of simple yoga every day has been shown to have demonstrable mental and physical benefits.

Yoga is built around a mind–body connection, which necessarily ensures a level of mindfulness. By refocusing the mind on the task at hand, by observing with pinpoint focus your breath, posture and balance, and by working towards achieving each pose in turn, and being very much present in that moment, there is little mental space for distracting thoughts. Yoga remains one of the best mental magnifying glasses, achieving a focused beam of thought, directed in a controlled and steady fashion.

GO FOR A WALK OR A RUN (PREFERABLY OUTSIDE!)

One of my favourite feelings is collapsing into bed in sheer physical exhaustion. The endorphin release that occurs during physical exercise delivers an instant lift of the mood, but long term has also been shown to help with depression – as has meditation. When huffing and puffing up a hill it is almost impossible not to be in that moment. The mind is singularly focused on the task of reaching the top. Every iota of consciousness is consumed by it, as moving becomes more strenuous. The chances are you will be very present, both emotionally and physically. That, in turn, takes you away from the cognitive stress of your daily life, helping to alleviate the impact of anxiety, which will leave you more receptive to sleep, and so more awake and focused during the day.

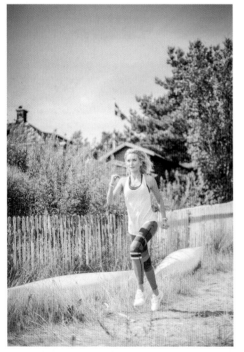

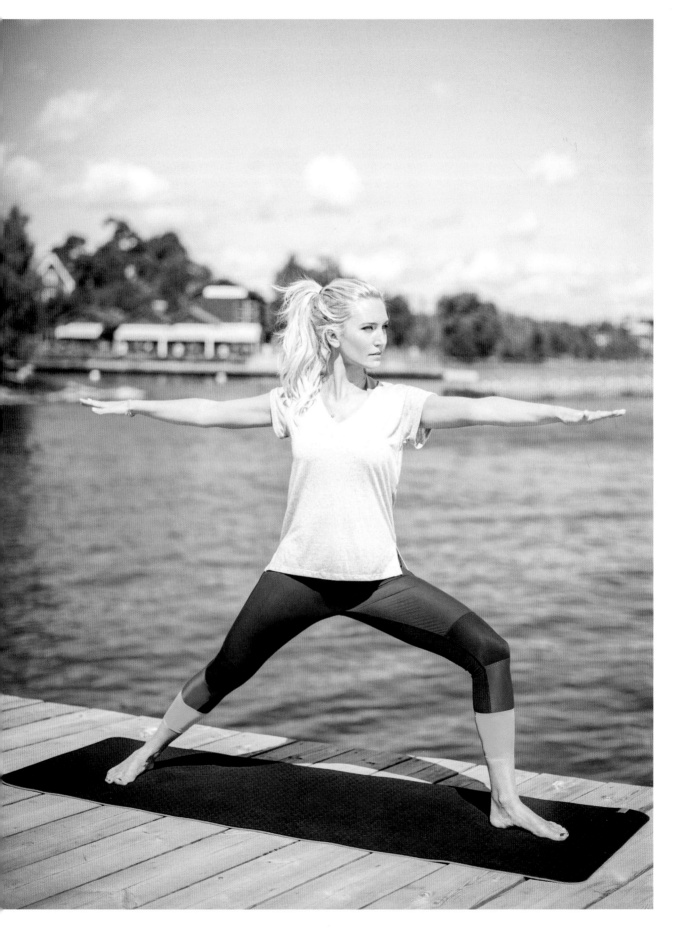

MINDFULNESS IN POSTURE AND MOVEMENT: SUN SALUTATION

The Sun Salutation is a classic yoga sequence in which one posture flows into the next in a continuous movement. It may take time to perfect, so don't worry if at first you seem to be stopping and starting. With practice the sequence will become second nature. Remember to breathe throughout (the little '+' symbol next to the illustrations means breathe in; '−' means breathe out). Listen to your body; if something hurts, adjust or stop.

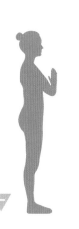

1 MOUNTAIN POSE

Standing tall with your feet together and your hands by your sides, roll your shoulders back and down, dropping them away from your ears. Focus on your breath, breathing in deeply through your nose and out through your mouth. Activate your abdominals by gently bringing your navel towards your spine. Root your feet into the floor and soften your knees. Lift your chest and tuck in your chin. Bring your palms together in front of your chest, fingers pointing upwards, as if in prayer. Exhale, preparing to flow into the standing backbend.

This pose is a chance to really quieten your thoughts and focus on your breath.

2 STANDING BACKBEND

Take a deep breath in and stretch your arms over your head, keeping your palms pressed together. Link your fingers and thumbs, keeping only your index fingers extended, as if pointing at the sky. Tip your head back and gaze up at your hands, lengthening your torso, keeping your abdominals engaged and creating a gentle arch in your back. Your chin should be in line with your arms. You can stop here, or if it feels comfortable, arch your back a little further, bringing your arms with the bend so that chin and arms stay aligned, and making sure your feet stay firmly planted on the floor. Hold the backbend for a moment, then return to standing.

This pose is a fabulous way to open out your chest and give the front of your body a good stretch.

3 FORWARD FOLD

Release your hands, but keep your arms up above you, then exhale and at the same time slowly and in a controlled manner roll your upper body downwards from the waist, drawing your navel in towards your spine. Fold your upper body over your thighs, keeping your legs straight but knees soft and letting your shoulders and head relax into the downward pull. Lay your palms flat on the floor, either side of your feet, fingers pointing forwards. Do not force it – bend your knees to enable your hands to lie flat, if you need to.

This is a fantastic pose for stretching out your hamstrings.

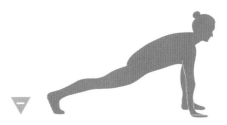

4 HALF LIFT

Inhale and lift your chest away from your thighs, sliding your hands up your feet and placing them on your shins. Keep your spine straight from your neck to your bottom. Look at the floor ahead of you.

5 LUNGE

Exhale and step your right foot back, bending your left knee and keeping your left shin upright and parallel with your arms, your left foot between your hands and creating a straight line from your right heel to the top of your head. Look at the floor, nose pointing downwards.

This is a fantastic stretch for your hip flexors.

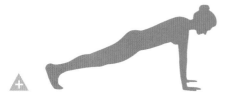

6 HIGH PLANK

Inhale and step your left foot back to meet your right, so that your feet are together. Keep your abs engaged the whole time. Form a straight line with your body, and ensure your arms are straight and your shoulders are over your hands.

This pose works your entire body and particularly your core (your back and abdominals).

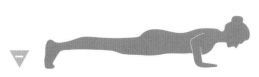

7 PUSH UP

Exhale and with control bend your elbows so that each arm forms a right angle, lowering your chest towards the floor. Keep your elbows tucked in and your body in a straight line. If you find this tricky, you can start by lowering your knees to the floor, raising your feet so that you're resting on your knees and then bending your elbows to form right angles and lowering your chest. (In this case lower your feet to the floor, toes tucked under, before you move on to the next step.)

This is a wonderful posture to strengthen your chest and arm muscles.

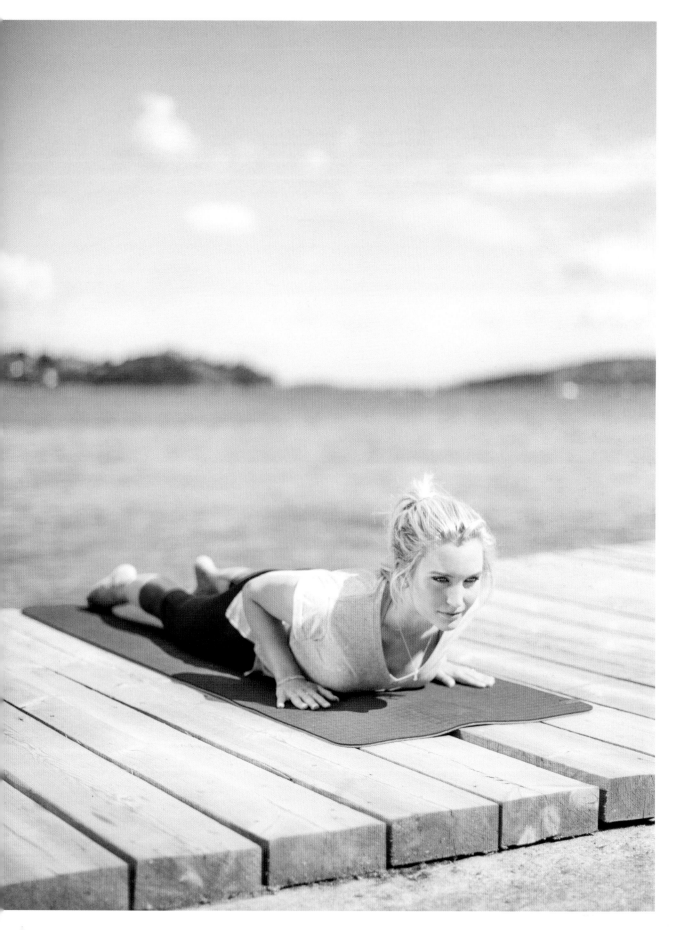

8 COBRA

Inhale and, keeping your hands and feet where they are, roll forwards onto the tops of your feet, roll your shoulders down and back, away from your ears, and try to bring your shoulder blades towards each other. Bring your chest between your straightened arms, open it out and tip your head back to gaze slightly upwards towards the sky. Gently squeeze your glutes. Hold this position for 1–3 breaths.

This is a great stretch for your abdominal muscles.

9 DOWNWARD DOG POSE

Engage your abdominals, exhale, and press into the floor, pushing your torso backwards and curling your toes under so that your feet are flat and your legs and your torso and arms create a triangle with the floor. Step your feet forwards, opening your legs and pointing your toes outwards to release the tension in your hamstrings. Press your palms into the floor to support your torso, spreading your fingers. Relax your head, making sure there's no tension in your neck or shoulders. Gaze between your arms towards your ankles behind you.

This pose strengthens your shoulders and provides a wonderful stretch for your back.

'One posture flows into the next in a continuous movement.'

10 REVERSE, THEN SWITCH SIDES

From Downward Dog, inhale and drop back down to Cobra, then roll back into Push Up, lift into High Plank, then bring yourself up into Half Lift. From here move into Forward Fold, then roll up one vertebra at time into Standing Backbend, and finally come back into Mountain Pose. Then, repeat the whole sequence (forwards and backwards), this time stepping your left foot back in Lunge (Step 5), so that you practise the sequence on the other side, too. This is important to keep your body in balance.

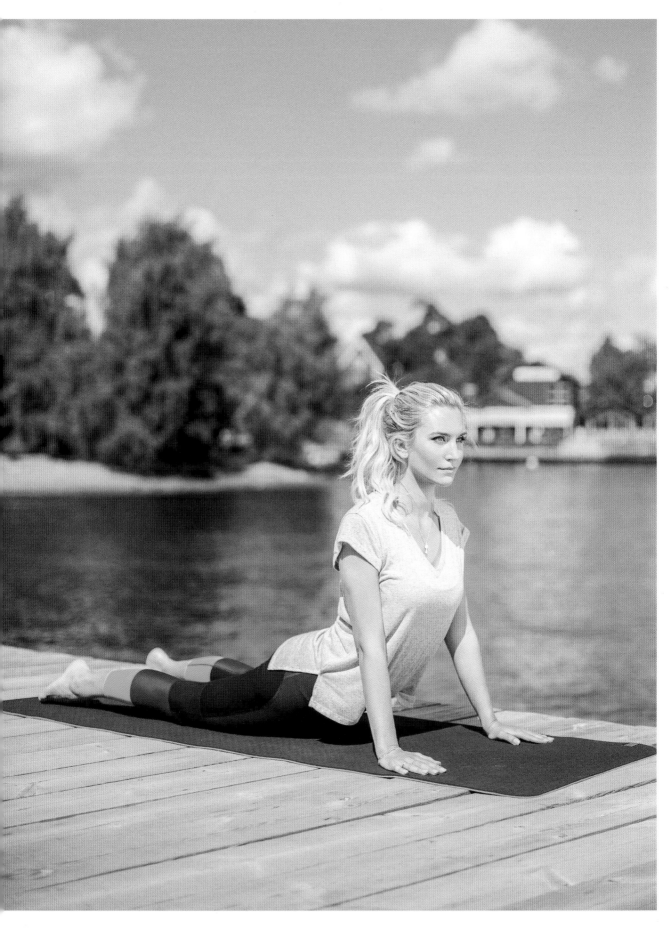

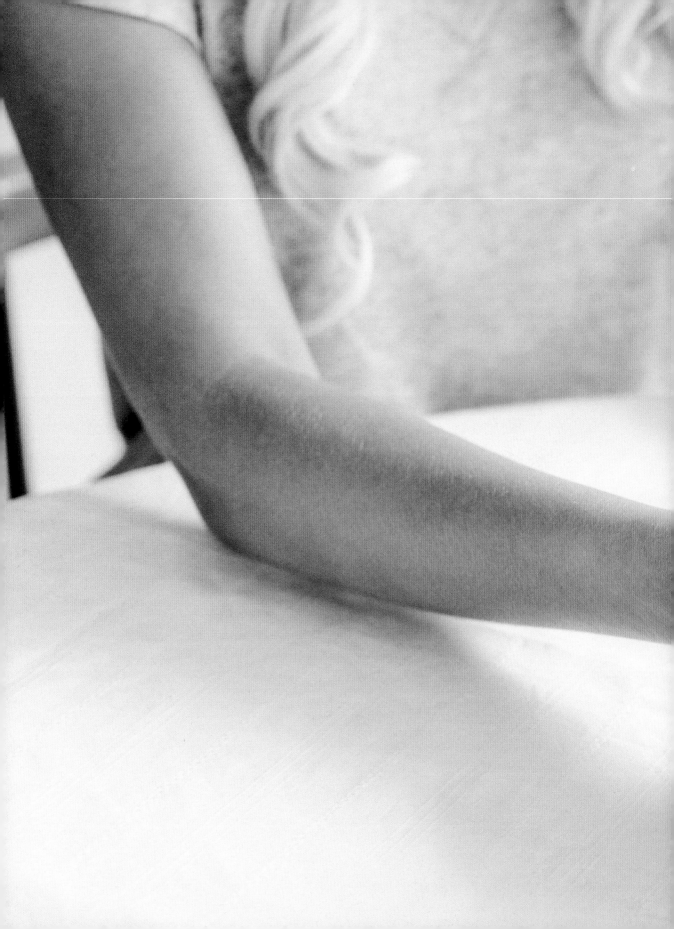

CHAPTER 2

Nourishing THE Body

'Healthy does not mean bland
or boring, but bursting with
varied flavour, and with exciting
tastes and textures.'

THE SCANDI ETHOS

Sweden has a bold and powerful cultural identity. You might have glimpsed morsels of my home nation's modern culture from our successful exports, like IKEA's revolutionary design, Abba's catchy music, Björn Borg's headbands – perhaps even the Swedish Chef from *Sesame Street* and his meatball fixation! But none of those speak to the underlying fabric of the Swedish – and, more broadly, Scandinavian – ethos. While there is no sacred scroll where our heritage is written down, it's passed along the generations through our upbringing – and especially through our food.

In Sweden there's still an intimate and deep connection to nature. For example, we mark the summer solstice, *Midsommar*, by dancing around the Maypole and decorating our houses with foliage. Above all, though, there's a devotion to an active, outdoorsy lifestyle – we value and respect the land and the sea alike. While that might all sound a bit foreign to you, the part that you can apply to everyday life is the national diet, which consists mainly of fresh, locally sourced, seasonal ingredients. That's what the recipes in this chapter will draw upon.

FISH, FISH AND MORE FISH

Crayfish, salmon, shrimp, lobster and herring are abundant in our waters and countless local dishes make great use of them. We even have an annual crayfish party, *Kräftskiva*, when we just go to town on boiled crayfish!

A PLACE TO FORAGE

In Sweden we have a concept called *allemansrätt*, literally meaning 'everyone's right' to walk freely on all lands, including private grounds. We use that freedom to seek out and pick fresh berries and fruits, as well as foraging for chanterelle and porcini mushrooms, which grow in abundance in our forests. You'll find plenty of recipes inspired by these freely available, natural resources.

'TIS THE SEASON

We cook in harmony with the seasons. Thanks to the long, harsh winters in Sweden, we have to make the most of what we have available, so many of our foods have historically been smoked or pickled, to make them last. We're a utilitarian bunch!

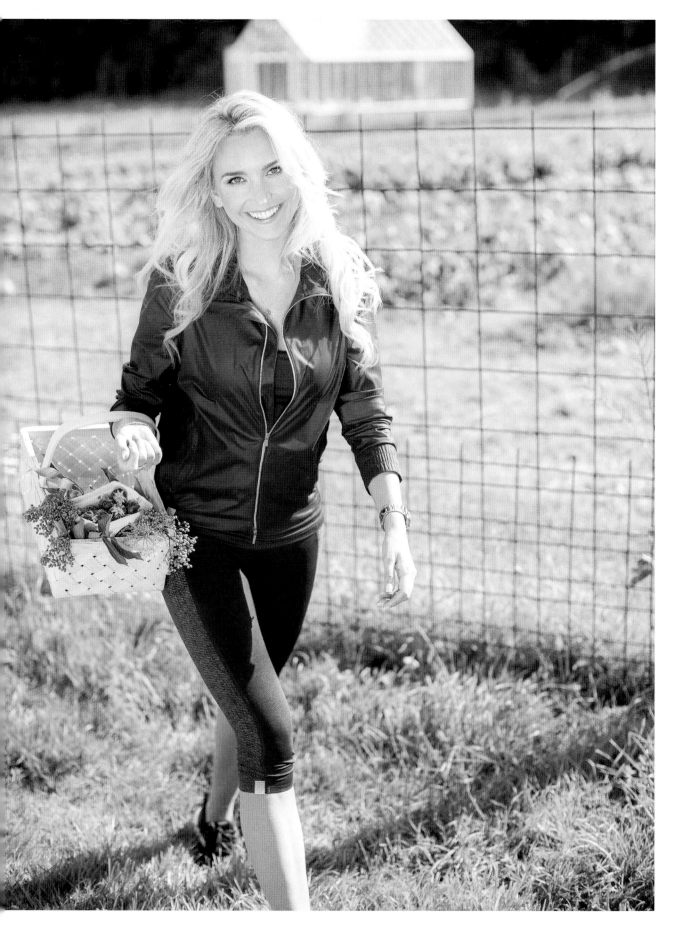

SMART FLAVOUR

The recipes you'll find in this section are intentionally loaded with what I call 'smart flavour' – plenty of spices and fresh herbs that are teeming with taste, but low in calories. Traditionally, Swedes use herbs such as dill and thyme for flavour, along with chives and garlic; we also make plentiful use of cinnamon, nutmeg and vanilla.

WASTE NOT, WANT NOT

We hate to waste! Making food in bulk is both time efficient and cost effective. Many of my recipes are safe to freeze, if you'd like, or to refrigerate and take to work as a packed lunch the following day. You won't find obscure ingredients that you have to source from high-end organic stores, but products you might find in your regular supermarket food aisle and that won't collect dust; you'll use them time and again.

WE TAKE OUR TIME

When having friends over, or indeed for those weekends when you're less time pressured, I've suggested some fish dishes that you can bake in the oven; they need a little more preparation and are ideally eaten hot. To cook in the kitchen can be such a meditative, relaxing experience. Occasionally, it's great just to take your time – a very Swedish pursuit!

THE CAKE OBSESSION!

It's not all savoury! The final part of my Scandi ethos, which is somewhat of a national institution, is *fika* – a Swedish word with no literal translation, but which in essence means 'to have a break, to drink a coffee with friends and enjoy a cake together'. I think it's a crucial part of anyone's healthy lifestyle that they feel liberated enough to indulge in what makes them happy. Demonising ingredients won't lead to a sustainable equilibrium, but everything in moderation most certainly will.

With that broad and balanced ethos in mind, I very much hope you enjoy making some or all of the Scandi-inspired recipes in this chapter! *Smaklig måltid* (*aka* bon appétit)!

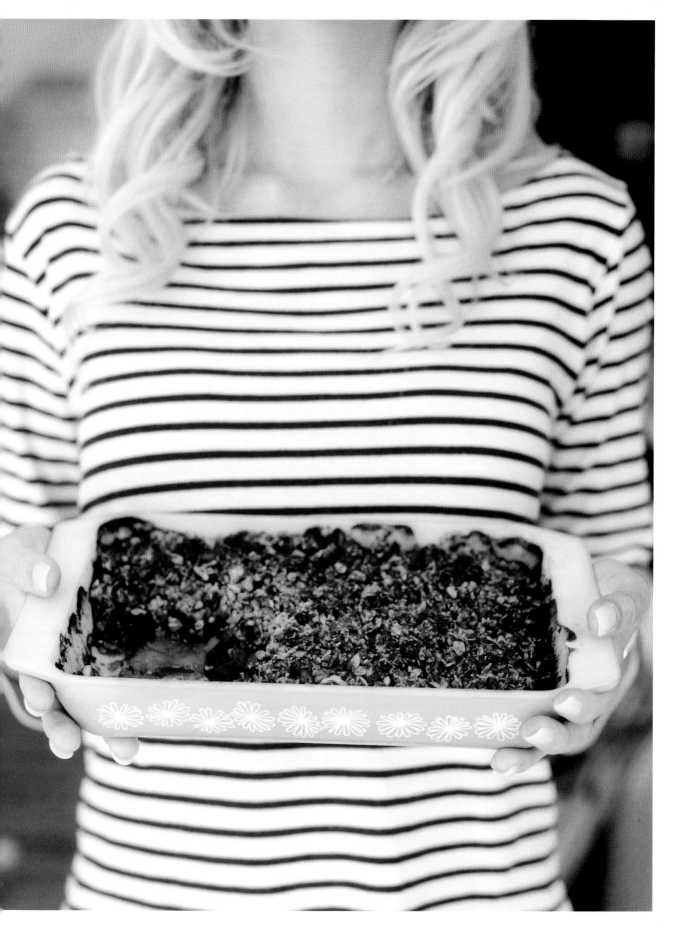

IT STARTS WITH DRINKING WATER

In Sweden, water is literally everywhere. We have more than 3,000km of coastline and, with the archipelago, too, there's just no getting away from it! And no drink delivers satisfaction like a glass of pure, ice-cold water – it fills you up, performs miracles for your skin and has a 0-calorie footprint! But given that water is a ubiquitous resource like air and sunlight, on average we simply don't get enough.

We lose 2.5 litres of water during the average day. We regain 1 litre through food and the remaining 1.5 litres are supposed to come from drinking water. Nobody likes a nag, but one of my consistent observations of those who struggle to 'get fit' is habitual dehydration; their bodies are operating in a permanent state of 'Gobi desert', which makes it really tough for the whole body to function properly.

WHAT IF YOU DON'T DRINK ENOUGH?

Dehydration is no laughing matter. Too little water can lead to light-headedness, fainting, headaches, fatigue and a loss of strength or stamina, and you might experience dryness of the skin around the lips, mouth and eyes. Your pulse may quicken, your immune system and metabolism may slow and you might struggle to concentrate. It's a groggy, uncomfortable, dream-like state.

SEVEN REASONS TO DRINK MORE

1 IMPROVE YOUR TRAINING Water helps deliver oxygen to your muscles to make them more efficient when you're working out. The more water inside the muscle cells, the better they're going to do their job. In the same way the giant redwood tree needs water to grow to such lofty heights and stay super-strong, so do we!

2 TRIM DOWN When we're dehydrated, we hold on to more available fluid, which can lead to bloating as well as weight gain. We retain extra water from any cells – including fat cells – in order to make up for the dehydration.

3 CLEAR YOUR HEAD If you're experiencing low energy levels, hunger or even headaches, you have the classic signs that you need to drink more. Instead of taking another paracetamol, or worse still wrongly identifying thirst as hunger (which will often lead to overeating), just try drinking a large glass of water – it's a superb natural appetite suppressant.

4 CHARGE UP YOUR METABOLISM Our kidneys are perfectly adapted to remove toxins. However, in a dehydrated body their filtration function just doesn't work so well and the poor liver has to work overtime! The liver's great at metabolising fat, but if it can't get that done efficiently, it can result in weight gain. Essentially, you're slowing down your organs, which means the whole system becomes slow, inefficient and lazy!

5 PURIFY THE BLOOD Almost 90 per cent of our bloodstream is water – making it a target for theft by a dehydrated body. If the body steals water from the blood, small capillaries close up, which thickens the blood and leaves you more prone to clots. What's the problem with that? Well, it tends to lead to hypertension, high cholesterol and heart disease – not exactly desirable!

6 SOAK IT UP Water can absorb and transport plenty of different nutrients found in food; it takes them on a journey along the digestive tract, and makes them more easily absorbable.

7 LOOSEN UP Water keeps your skin, eyes and mouth hydrated as well as providing natural lubrication to your muscles and joints, which significantly reduces the risk of sprains or cramp, enabling you to lift heavier, a little bit easier.

A WORD OF WARNING!

Drinking water means drinking *water*. Pure and simple. Don't try to cheat your way to your daily quota with juices, squash, alcohol, or caffeine or energy drinks. Recently, I bumped into a friend at the gym who'd just smashed out an hour-long workout and then downed a 1-litre bottle of shop-bought, fruit-flavoured 'water'. Little did she know she'd just guzzled ten teaspoons of liquid sugar! The moral of the story: *ignorance is remiss*! The exception to pure water will please all you keen tea drinkers, but make sure you stick to the decaffeinated kind (ideally, herbal or fruit teas). Cups of caffeine-free tea add up and help keep you hydrated.

HOW TO MAKE IT A BIT MORE INTERESTING...

On a normal day, I drink about 2 litres of water. A trick I like to use is to mark up a 2-litre bottle in ten equally spaced increments, then label them 8am, 9am, 10am and so on, using a permanent marker. As we can absorb only around 200ml of water per hour, that's an easy and smart way to ensure you stay on top of it! Here are some of my favourite flavoursome tricks to help ease the monotony of drinking more:

▶ Water with cucumber
▶ Water with strawberries and lime
▶ Water with lemon
▶ Water with orange slices
▶ Water with blueberries and raspberries
▶ Water with ginger
▶ Water with fresh mint leaves

YOUR THREE NUTRITIONAL FRIENDS: CARBS, FATS AND PROTEIN

All the foods you eat fall broadly into one of three 'macronutrient' camps: carbohydrates (carbs), fats and protein. All three are *essential* sources of energy and nourishment, but you can guarantee that at any one time, a popular diet will be demonising one of them. I believe in a balanced approach, as all three macronutrients are beneficial in the right quantities; cutting out entire food groups is simply not sustainable or particularly healthy. I regularly overhear gym-goers discussing a wacky diet they're trying out, whether it's juice-cleansing, starving for two days a week, protein-bingeing or an online purchase that 'guarantees' you'll 'lose X kg in less than Y weeks'. Any plan that claims cutting out a complete food group is a good idea sets alarm bells ringing for me. To cut something out entirely often results in a very limited (and boring) diet, and in my opinion just isn't necessary.

CARBOHYDRATES
General rule: 1g of carbohydrate will provide 4 calories of energy.

Many people think of 'carby' food only in terms of starch-heavy items like white pasta and bread and potatoes. It's important to know, however, that apples and broccoli also contain carbohydrate.

Low-GI, 'complex' carbohydrates (such as whole grains, wholewheat bran and pasta, and brown rice, among others) release energy (glucose) into your bloodstream slowly, sustaining you throughout the day. On the other hand, high-GI, 'simple' carbs (white pasta and bread, fizzy drinks and so on) turn you into a hyper two-year-old for an hour, then comatose you for the next five. Eating more complex carbs leaves you less peckish and gives you energy for longer! It's important to eat carbohydrates post-workout, mainly to replenish the muscles' stores of glycogen, which you've burned through during your workout. Refuelled, your muscles can repair and work even better next time!

FATS
General rule: 1g of fat will provide 9 calories of energy.

Good fats work wonders for your skin, hair, training results and general wellbeing. You don't need to skip fats to lose weight – the body *needs* them for a range of functions, such as:

▸ Growth and repair of tissue, including muscle cells.

▸ Absorption of fat-soluble vitamins, such as vitamins A, D, E and K, which can become deficient in a low-fat diet.

▸ Cushioning organs and insulating nerve cells.

▸ Facilitating your body's temperature control (thermoregulation).

Of course, you should avoid *some* fats – trans fatty acids, for example. Also known simply as trans fats, they're not naturally occurring, but are artificially concocted through a process called 'hydrogenation' – converting liquid fat to solid. They're often found in margarines, cakes, biscuits and junk food in general, and they increase the unhealthy cholesterol (HDL) in your body and reduce the good type (LDL). They are proven to increase your risk of coronary heart disease, stroke, high blood pressure and more.

By contrast, monounsaturated fat is a 'good' fat. It can be found naturally in olive oil, nuts, avocados and some seeds. It can lower your blood cholesterol and decrease your risk of heart disease. Polyunsaturated fat also falls into the 'good' column, and mainly derives from plants, vegetable oil, nuts and oily fish. Essential

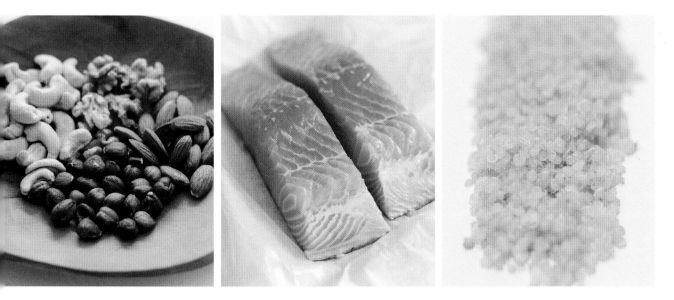

fatty acids, such as omega-3 (found in foods such as wild salmon, edamame, walnuts and flax seed) and omega-6 (vegetable oil, black beans and wild rice), are polyunsaturated fats. We call them 'essential' because we have to obtain them from our food. Generally speaking, if a fat is naturally occurring, in moderation it'll be useful to your body's operation.

PROTEIN

General rule: 1g of protein provides 4 calories of energy.

Protein is a super-important part of any balanced diet. In the weights zone of the gym, it's often worshipped for its 'growth and repair' (or 'get huge') properties, but it regulates many other body functions, too – including digestion, absorption, blood oxygenation, bone strength, antibody production, brain activity and even fingernail regeneration!

Amino acids are the building blocks of protein and are found in a variety of foods. Meat, milk, cheese and egg are 'complete' proteins that have all the essential amino acids. Other sources of protein include beans, legumes, peas and peanut butter. For those who do not eat meat, eggs or dairy products, it is important to eat a variety of these other foods to clock up the amino acids. You don't typically associate high protein with vegetables, but certain grains and seeds are incredibly rich in protein. Quinoa is one of them, and its carbohydrate content is sufficiently low-GI/slow-release to make it the ultimate ingredient to complement your healthy lifestyle.

How much is the right amount of protein? It's thought that the average adult who's just 'ticking over' should consume 0.79g for every kilo of body weight. Elite athletes may be able to process three times this number, but the normal human who's training as part of a healthy lifestyle might use this 0.79g as a base guide, and take it from there. Eating more protein doesn't necessarily mean more or better repair, as there's a limit to what the body can do in a given period of time, so keep this in mind!

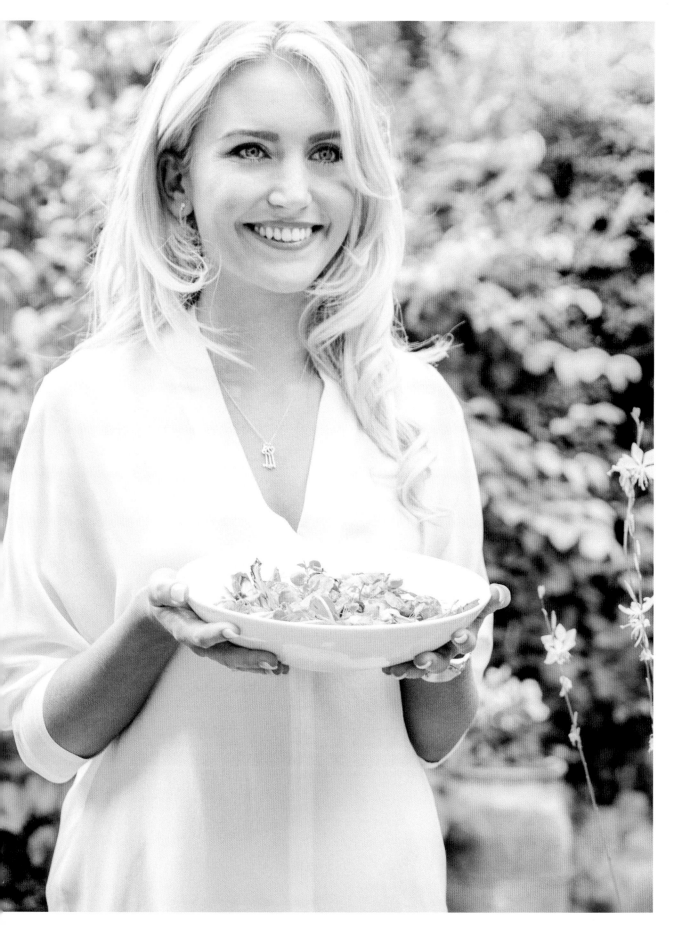

WHAT IS A GDA?

GDA stands for Guideline Daily Amount, the amount of a certain nutrient the UK Government recommends for a balanced diet in a healthy adult. It's a bit of a blunt tool: it won't account for your age, size or lifestyle, so take the following with a pinch of salt (literally!) – but at least they give a decent steer.

FAT
The adult GDA is around 70g, of which saturates (which are unhealthy fats) are 20g. If, on the label's 'per 100g' column, the product has over 20 per cent overall fats, I tend to be cautious. I'll also consider a product truly 'low fat' if the fats figure is sub 5 per cent.

SUGAR
The adult GDA is around 90g. Sugar is a form of carbohydrate, so keep an eye on the 'Carbohydrates (of which sugars)' part of the label, too. I try to opt for complex carbohydrates, which release energy slowly to sustain blood sugar at a steadier rate through the day – whole wheat, whole grains, pulses, seeds and nuts. Too much simple 'refined' sugar can lead to risk of diabetes, high blood pressure and heart disease.

SALT
The adult GDA is around 6g, just over one teaspoon! We need salt to regulate fluid balance in the body, but too much of it, over too long a time frame, can lead to problems such as stroke, high blood pressure and heart disease. I like to substitute salt with alternative flavour enhancers, such as herbs and spices, or a squeeze of lemon juice. If you buy tinned fish, get the 'in spring water' option rather than 'in brine', and watch out for salty sauces, too!

CALORIES
The adult GDA is around 2000 kcal (calories) a day, but a truer reflection would vary significantly depending on gender, activity levels and your metabolic condition. Calories are a measure of the amount of energy contained within your food, and we don't need to demonise them, but, rather, understand them. Eat too much energy, and you'll store the unused excess as fat; eat too little and you'll supplement the deficit by dipping into your fat reserves. I don't like to focus too much on the total number of calories per se, but it's helpful for measuring 'energy in' versus 'energy out'. It's all about the balance!

FOOD LABELS ARE ESSENTIAL READING

How do you know what's in each food you eat? All the packaged foods you buy have a label that the law says must give you a clear analysis of what you're eating. In practice, your blueberry milkshake might not actually contain any blueberries, much as your cheese-and-onion crisps probably don't contain cheese. Or onion. Reading the food labels will help you to see what's going in.

Awareness and healthy cynicism are important, too. Often the word 'light' will be thrown into the equation, to help cajole you into thinking you're buying a diet product. There is no official definition of 'light' and in reality it may simply be 'lighter' than another comparable product (though who knows which one?). Likewise, there's no official definition of 'low fat', so a curious mind that reads the label, weighs up the percentages and puts it into the context of the GDA (see box, opposite) will quickly learn to read between the lines. Don't let the food producer insult your intelligence, and don't be too quick to trust all marketing claims!

BEWARE WHAT'S ON TOP

The nearer the top of an ingredient list a certain ingredient appears, the more of it there is in that food compared with the other ingredients. So, if honey is the third ingredient on a twenty-strong list, as natural as honey is, that's a lot of sugar!

COMPARE AND CONTRAST – KEEP IT SIMPLE!

If Product A contains 20g fat per 100g, that's 20 per cent fat; if the product weighs 200g and you scoff the whole thing, then that's 40g of fat you just put away. Your GDA is 70g, so that's almost 60 per cent of your daily ideal. Quite a lot. However, if Product B has 10g fat per 100g, and weighs 200g, then you're consuming 20g of fat; closer to 30 per cent of your GDA. In this example, Product B would clearly be the lighter choice. There are complexities around the type of fat, too, and indeed types of sugar, but the decision process between products should be a question of simple maths!

USING YOUR LABEL KNOW-HOW

When I read a food label, I usually have four concerns:

1 Is this food high in fat?
2 Is it high in saturates?
3 Is it high in sugar?
4 Is it high in salt?

A suite of yeses won't necessarily mean a rejection (see page 38 for more on treating yourself!), but I do follow it up with one more question: is it worth it? That, of course, comes down to a judgement about whether the delicious cinnamon bun justifies you spending, say, 30 per cent of your daily sugar 'budget' and 25 per cent of your daily fat 'wallet' on one parcel of deliciousness. It might well make the cut, but understanding food labels just means you are able to make an informed decision.

A WORD ON ALCOHOL

There are a host of Scandinavian festivals that revolve around (responsible, *ahem!*) drinking and I enjoy a tipple as much as the next Swede! But if you're trying to improve your overall health, it's important to remember that alcoholic drinks are brimming with sugars and empty calories; they offer no nutritional benefit and encourage weight gain. Nobody wants to live a life of relentless, monk-like restraint, but an awareness of what's in alcohol can help you to manage portion control.

IF YOU MUST...

Make it a glass of red. Research shows that red wine may boost good cholesterol and so decrease the risk of stroke and heart disease. It's also rich in certain polyphenol antioxidants, which help with cell health. Or, I opt for spirits (such as vodka, gin or Scotch) with ice. I avoid mixers, which are bursting with simple sugars.

IN SHORT...

A night out involving three or four drinks – followed by some cheesy chips! – could easily amount to 1250 to 1500 calories, which is potentially around 70 per cent of your daily allowance! It's no wonder that the next day you'll feel bloated and tired. Having said all that, the occasional lychee martini is fine – and if it provides a reward for a week of good work, which keeps you on track with your overall health goals, I'm all for it!

KEEP SCORE

This table gives you a basic guide to the number of calories and the amount of sugar (and how much sugar that equates to in terms of the GDA for adults) in certain measures and types of alcohol.

ALCOHOL	MEASURE	CALORIES	SUGAR
Double gin + tonic	250ml	150 kcal	18g, or 4 teaspoons (25% of your GDA)
Champagne	120ml	91 kcal	2g, or about ½ teaspoon (about 4% of your GDA)
Lager	440ml	247 kcal	8g, or 2 teaspoons (about 13% of your GDA)
Vodka	35ml	55 kcal	Sugar-free!
Baileys	125ml	409 kcal	25g, or 6 teaspoons (36% of your GDA)
Rum + regular cola	250ml	129 kcal	28g, or 7 teaspoons (40% of your GDA)
Wine (14% ABV)	250ml	230 kcal	2g sugar, or about ½ teaspoon (about 4% of your GDA)

A WORD ON SUGAR

Sugar is a popular demon these days, blamed for any number of health issues. Some of those claims might be true, but not all sugars are created equal! A form of carbohydrate, sugar provides raw energy for our bodies. We need it to power our furnaces – that is, to live!

I try to avoid sugars that are refined, processed, simple or 'high-GI' (see p.42). They serve no nutritional purpose and are absorbed into the bloodstream ultra-quickly, causing blood-sugar levels to rocket, then crash, leaving you zombified and hungry again. You'll find refined sugars in sweets, fizzy drinks, white bread and rice, and processed foods containing high fructose corn syrup. A good rule of thumb: *if it tastes too sweet, it probably is*! The mortal enemies (and my close friends) of 'bad' sugars are low-GI, complex sugars, which are more slowly absorbed into the bloodstream, stabilising energy levels. You'll find them in products such as wholegrain and wholewheat foods, sweet potatoes, and porridge oats. Eating complex sugars means that you don't feel peaks and troughs of hunger as much, and feel more energised more of the time!

Entire books have been written on sugar, but my view is simple: be aware, know what to look for on the label (see box, right), know how much you're consuming, and know what type you're consuming. If it's something you can identify as lower-GI, is natural and contains a limited total amount of sugar, it's probably a good way to nourish your body with the energy it needs.

TREATING YOURSELF

I love chocolate. Always have, always will. I believe chocolate is *essential*. If I incorporate a modest amount of chocolate into my training diet, it is no longer taboo and I get to enjoy that delicious moment of dopamine release (*aka* happiness!). You have to embrace the things that make you happy; you get only one shot at life. Now, chocolate might not float your boat, but everyone has their 'thing'. By allowing yourself that thing, in moderation on a regular basis, you're more likely to stay on the straight and narrow the rest of the time. Obviously be sensible about amounts – a whole 500g bar of chocolate isn't a 'modest' amount, but a few squares of 70-per-cent dark chocolate will do the 'treat' job very nicely. Enjoy!

SYNONYMS FOR SUGAR

The following list of names for 'sugar' is by no means exhaustive, but it will give you a good start on what to look for – and to avoid in excess – when you're reading food labels:

- ▶ maltose
- ▶ dextrose
- ▶ sucrose
- ▶ high-fructose
- ▶ corn syrup
- ▶ anything followed by 'sweetener'

And, remember, the higher up the ingredient list sugar appears, the more sugar that food product contains.

YOUR NUTRITION IN PRACTICE

Over the years, I've pored over countless pages of clients' food diaries and I've observed some common themes; the practicalities of good nutrition that come up time and again. They're things that I *know* people want and need, and that help them stick to their goals. I wanted to ensure all these observations were a part of each recipe in *Fit in 3*!

SPICE UP YOUR LIFE

Not only will spices give your food a rich, full flavour, they'll deliver potent health benefits, too, including disease-fighting antioxidants and protection against chronic conditions (such as cancers, diabetes and heart disease). They're packed with vitamins and minerals and remarkably low in calories. Try chilli powder to boost your metabolism, cinnamon for its restorative properties, and curry leaves, ginger or turmeric to boost your iron levels. On the herb side, favourites are fresh basil, parsley, coriander and lemongrass. Pop into your local grocer and start experimenting with these little giants of super-healthy flavour!

QUICK AND EASY!

Whether or not people love to cook, the one thing they all have in common is time; or, the lack of it. Each recipe in this book is quick and easy to make. The core recipes are designed to be assembled by a complete novice in the kitchen. Why? Because fresh produce is so delicious and wholesome by itself that it needs few ornamental frills; fresh tuna steak, organic avocado… these are uncomplicated foods that simply don't benefit from culinary complication!

ACCESSIBLE, REUSABLE AND AFFORDABLE

In general, people value convenience, and that means *not* having to source obscure, exotic and costly ingredients; ingredients that may get used only once or twice and thereafter collect dust or go out of date. In this book the recipe ingredients are practical; you'll find them in your local supermarket's food aisles; you'll use them again and again so they're worth buying in bulk. The recipes will show you how a host of the same ingredients can have several different flavour outcomes! More importantly, the recipes are eminently affordable to make and aim to show that eating healthily shouldn't be difficult and doesn't need to cost a fortune.

IT SHOULD TASTE GOOD!

Healthy does *not* mean bland or boring, but bursting with varied flavour; exciting tastes and textures. It will leave you feeling full and satisfied. Many of my clients have bad memories of 'groundhog meals' – endless steamed broccoli, lean chicken breasts and protein shakes. Using a host of herbs and spices, my recipes are loaded with flavour without being loaded with empty calories.

IT MUST BE BALANCED

The fitness industry is awash with commercialised 'superfoods', 'smoothies' and 'protein snacks'; they're brilliantly marketed,

15 TIPS FOR HEALTHY EATING

1   Befriend your local butcher or fishmonger – opt for local produce where possible, not just for its environmental impact, but also its freshness and superior taste.

2   Always read the label and digest the pros and cons, before you proceed to digest them for real!

3   Roast, bake, grill or steam, but avoid frying as often as you can.

4   Make in bulk, then store away for the remainder of the week. Healthy eating then becomes easily accessible when the urge for food takes you.

5   Eat a variety of foods that you enjoy, or else you're risking 'clean fatigue' and you'll end up bingeing!

6   Portion control matters – avoid overeating and eat only when you're hungry.

7   Remember, you may be thirsty, not hungry – drink plenty of water throughout the day.

8   Chew your food well – it breaks it down and improves your digestion.

9   Eat slowly and in a relaxed environment to give your brain time to recognise when you're full.

10 Use less salt in your cooking and avoid high-sodium foods. Delicious fresh, natural food shouldn't need to rely on salt for flavour, and your heart will thank you for it.

11 Eat lots of raw fruits and vegetables, which are more nutritionally intact than cooked versions.

12 Keep your food simple and quick – it's a guarantee that you'll stick to your healthy diet.

13 Eat regularly – it will help keep your blood-sugar levels stable so that you don't risk high-sugar snacks.

14 Make healthy eating your routine: remember that even if you miss a meal or slip up now and again, if most of what you're eating is clean, fresh and nutritious, you'll soon get right back on track.

15 Dedicate at least one meal a week to indulge in one of your favourite foods, whether that be pizza or American pancakes. It helps to anchor you and keep you sane.

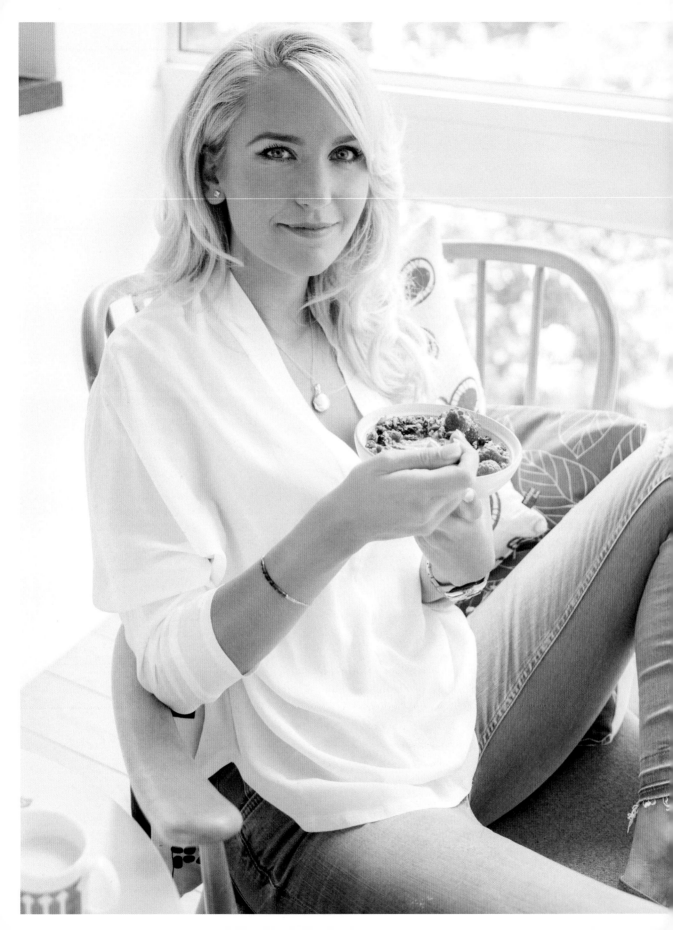

but one has to ask what is in fact healthy, and what's just cleverly disguised. In this book, every recipe has been looked over by a professional nutritionist to ensure balance. The recipes provide:

- ▸ low levels of sodium
- ▸ low levels of saturated fat
- ▸ a balance of protein, fat and carbohydrate
- ▸ low levels of refined sugar

You'll find a list giving you macro-nutrient content at the top of each recipe, and each has a series of icons to tell you if it's gluten-free, dairy-free and/or vegetarian (see panel, bottom right). Bear in mind that some dairy-free recipes will need you to take the dairy-free milk or yogurt option in the ingredients. It is also worth noting here that portion size is for an average-sized, healthy adult – the limitations of print mean that, sadly, I can't tailor to your uniqueness. While the recipes are nutritionally balanced it's up to you to determine the right portion size for you.

THE SCANDINAVIAN TWIST?

I remember some of these recipes very fondly, as I grew up with them during my childhood in Sweden. Others I've developed to help you benefit from a specific Scandinavian nuance or influence. All of them draw upon the healthiest aspects of Swedish eating (see pp. 36–8), and all honour the Scandinavian tradition of using fresh, local produce, and flavouring foods with spices and fresh herbs.

MORE FISH!

While I'm a pescatarian and have been since the age of eight, it's not something I enforce on others. Having said that, I know that it's not unusual to encounter individuals who rarely eat any fish at all, which is a shame as it's an exceptional source of lean protein and omega-3 and -6 fatty acids (see pp.42–4) – and there's so much you can do with it. For these reasons there are more fish recipes than there are meat recipes in this book. That's also reflective of the Swedish national diet; we're blessed with thousands of kilometres of ocean border, so in Sweden we know a thing or two about fishing! Also, it's a bit cold for most cows.

NUTRITION IN THE THREE-WEEK PLAN

Chapter Four sets out a three-week plan for wellness, including, for each day, a nutritionally balanced food plan based on the recipes on pages 54–137. Every day you'll find a suggestion for a morning juice shot, a breakfast, a lunch and a dinner, as well as snacks for mid-morning and mid-afternoon. I've also harnessed the idea of meat-free Monday – the first day of each week in the plan is meat-free! Overall, I've designed the menus to be flexible, to reflect how people like to live their lives. Feel free to swap around meals as you go, if you like. If you want to swap day one's lunch for day three's lunch – then go ahead! That's OK!

KEY TO RECIPE ICONS

GF Gluten-free

DF Dairy-free

V Vegetarian

BREAKFASTS

There's a reason why so many people call breakfast the most important meal of the day. A good breakfast will underpin that day's eating patterns, helping you to settle into a stable dietary rhythm. You'll be less likely to suffer a mid-morning bout of ravenous hunger, causing a panicked scramble for food... which in turn will have the same effect mid-afternoon and again in the evening! Many of the breakfast recipes in this section are time-savers you can make in bulk and roll out as you wish – each one setting you up for a busy day ahead. But come the weekend, or any day when you have a little extra time in the morning, there's also a handful of delicious breakfast treats, to make this vital meal extra special!

QUINOA GRANOLA

1 portion gives you ▶ FAT 20.6g (of which SATURATES 4.9g) ▶ CARBOHYDRATE 21.5g (of which SUGARS 8.9g) ▶ FIBRE 1.8g ▶ PROTEIN 8g ▶ SALT 0.02g

Based upon the zeitgeist superfood 'quinoa' (pronounced *kin-wah*), here's my granola – a splendid breakfast offering, loaded with nutritional value and a sweet taste to satisfy the morning sugar craving. Supermarket granola tends to be a hiding place for simple sugars and transfats, but my homemade edition is altogether more healthy. Oats are out, quinoa is in[-wah], and a host of cinnamon-covered nuts and seeds make a guest appearance. Rather than demonising sweetness, I've lightly glazed the granola with natural Manuka honey.

SERVES 6–8

PREP TIME: **15 minutes**

COOKING TIME: **25 minutes**

125g (4½oz) quinoa

40g (1½oz) almonds, coarsely chopped

40g (1½oz) hazelnuts, coarsely chopped

40g (1½oz) pecans, coarsely chopped

40g (1½oz) sunflower seeds

40g (1½oz) pumpkin seeds

1 heaped tbsp coconut oil

1 heaped tbsp good-quality raw honey

1 tbsp ground cinnamon

60g (2¼oz) dried unsweetened cherries, cranberries or raisins

2 tbsp shelled hemp seeds (optional)

plain live yogurt or dairy-free alternative, fresh berries and/or unsweetened Homemade Almond Milk (see p.136), or milk of choice, to serve

Pour the quinoa into a small saucepan, cover with water and bring to the boil. Turn the heat down, cover with the lid and simmer for 5 minutes – you want the grains to soften slightly but not become too soft and mushy. Drain the quinoa well, then spread it out on a clean tea towel to cool and drain.

Heat the oven to 180°C/350°F/Gas Mark 4 and line two baking trays with baking paper.

Tip the quinoa into a mixing bowl and stir in the nuts and seeds.

Gently heat the coconut oil and honey together in a small pan, then pour it over the quinoa mixture. Add the cinnamon and stir well until everything is mixed together.

Spread out the mixture on the baking trays and toast in the oven for 17–20 minutes, or until everything smells toasted and the quinoa has crisped up. Halfway through cooking, swap the trays round in the oven and turn the granola mixture so it cooks evenly.

Tip the granola into a bowl and leave it to cool and crisp up further. Stir in the dried fruit and hemp seeds, if using. When completely cold, transfer the granola to a jar.

There are lots of different ways to serve the granola but I like to spoon some yogurt into a bowl, sprinkle the granola over the top and finish it with a handful of fresh berries. (I also like the granola with almond milk, which works perfectly, too.)

MAX MUESLI

1 portion gives you ▶ FAT **32.7g** (of which SATURATES **4.6g**) ▶ CARBOHYDRATE **43.7g** (of which SUGARS **7.8g**)
▶ FIBRE **7.1g** ▶ PROTEIN **15g** ▶ SALT **0.04g**

I don't joke about muesli; it's a very serious subject! A core component of my weekly nutrition (when it's the homemade kind, of course – supermarket muesli lacks natural authenticity… trust me), it's a super-easy breakfast that teems with essential vitamins and minerals to nourish me for the day ahead. One weekend day each fortnight, I try to mix up a batch to last me the two weeks. I'll empty the key ingredients into a plastic cereal container, close the lid and shake it around vigorously (great cardio). Then I'm ready to dispatch a serving whenever breakfast time arrives.

SERVES **7**

PREP TIME: **10 minutes, plus soaking**

COOKING TIME: **6 minutes**

70g (2½oz) walnut halves

70g (2½oz) almonds

280g (10oz) sugar-free puffed wholegrain brown rice or puffed spelt flakes, or jumbo porridge oats

70g (2½oz) Brazil nuts, roughly chopped

100g (3½oz) sunflower seeds

3 tbsp ground flaxseeds

3 tbsp shelled hemp seeds

100g (3½oz) dried unsulphured apricots, roughly chopped

chia seeds, unsweetened Homemade Almond Milk (see p.136), or milk of choice, ground cinnamon and blueberries, to serve

First toast the nuts – you can roast them in the oven but if you're only toasting a small amount it makes sense to do this on the hob. Put the walnuts in a large, dry frying pan and toast them over a medium-low heat for 3 minutes, turning once, until they start to colour. Tip them into a bowl and leave to cool while you repeat this with the almonds.

Once they are cool, roughly chop the walnuts and almonds, then tip them into a bowl with the puffed cereal, Brazil nuts, sunflower seeds, flaxseeds and hemp seeds. Stir in the apricots until everything is mixed together.

If serving with chia seeds, soak them in almond milk in a bowl for a minimum of 15 minutes (or you can leave them overnight). Top the chia with a serving of muesli, your favourite milk, a sprinkling of cinnamon and a final topping of blueberries.

APPLE & DATE MIXED GRAIN PORRIDGE

1 portion gives you ▶ FAT **4.4g** (of which SATURATES **1.7g**) ▶ CARBOHYDRATE **50.9g** (of which SUGARS **14.1g**) ▶ FIBRE **3.7g** ▶ PROTEIN **6.8g** ▶ SALT **0.2g**

Swedes are notoriously anti-waste; we just hate to let good stuff go in the bin. One risky candidate is often a six- or eight-pack of apples (unless you're munching one or more a day, of course). So, any leftover apples about to go off? Porridge to the rescue! This sumptuous little recipe is hugely reminiscent of a Swedish breakfast I used to eat before trudging through the snowy blizzards to school. A classic dish that packs a refuelling punch, it also satisfies the sweeter tooth and sustains you right through to lunch (or at least until breaktime).

SERVES **2**

PREP TIME: **10 minutes**

COOKING TIME: **10 minutes**

100g (3½oz) mixed flaked grains such as oat, quinoa, amaranth and buckwheat or your grain of choice

300ml (10½fl oz) unsweetened Homemade Almond Milk (see p.136), or milk of choice

ground cinnamon, for sprinkling

toasted nuts and seeds of choice, to serve

APPLE & DATE MUSH

1 apple, skin-on, grated and core discarded

2 pitted dates, chopped

squeeze of lemon juice

Put the grains and milk in a saucepan with 400ml (14fl oz) water and bring to the boil over a medium heat, stirring well.

Turn the heat down to low and simmer for 10 minutes, stirring with a wooden spoon, or until the grains are tender and creamy. Add a splash more milk or water if you need to.

While the porridge is cooking, make the apple and date mush. Put the apple in a small pan with the dates, lemon juice and 2–3 tablespoons water. Cook over a medium-low heat for 6–8 minutes, covered with the lid and stirring often, until the fruit is very soft and mushy. Mash the apple mixture with the back of a fork until almost smooth.

Spoon the porridge into bowls, swirl in the apple mush or spoon it on top. Sprinkle with cinnamon and finish with some toasted nuts and seeds.

SUNDAE FOR SUNDAY

1 portion gives you ▶ FAT **13.9g** (of which SATURATES **2.2g**) ▶ CARBOHYDRATE **23.4g** (of which SUGARS **10.5g**)
▶ FIBRE **5.6g** ▶ PROTEIN **10.3g** ▶ SALT **0.14g**

This is what I like to think of as a Jedi 'mind-trick' dish — something that looks and practically tastes like a dessert, but in reality is a nutritionally dependable breakfast. It's loaded with chia seeds, which are part of the superfood élite and practically defy the laws of physics. Yes, each seed is miniature, but its superpowers are outsized. Chia seeds expand by nine times when in water (keeping you fuller for longer), they're antioxidant rich, and a wonderful source of protein and healthy fats (eight times more than salmon!). Furthermore, they're great for the skin, hair and nails!

SERVES **2**

PREP TIME: **15 minutes, plus soaking**

COOKING TIME: **5 minutes**

½ ripe papaya or mango, cut in
  half, seeds or stone removed,
  peeled and diced
1 tbsp chia seeds
2 tbsp jumbo porridge oats
2 tbsp flaked almonds
8 tbsp unsweetened coconut or
  plain live yogurt
a few blueberries and ground
  cinnamon, to serve

Put three-quarters of the papaya or mango in a small blender with 2–3 tablespoons of water and blend until smooth. Pour the purée into a bowl and gently stir in the chia seeds. Leave the chia seeds to swell and thicken the purée for at least an hour, or preferably overnight in the fridge.

Meanwhile, put the oats and almonds in a large, dry frying pan and toast them over a medium-low heat for 2–3 minutes, tossing the pan frequently, until they smell toasted and start to colour. Tip them onto a plate and leave them to cool.

Divide half of the oat mixture between two glasses or small bowls, spoon over the papaya or mango mixture and the yogurt. Just before serving, top with the remaining diced papaya or mango, the blueberries, the remaining toasted oat mixture and finally a sprinkling of cinnamon.

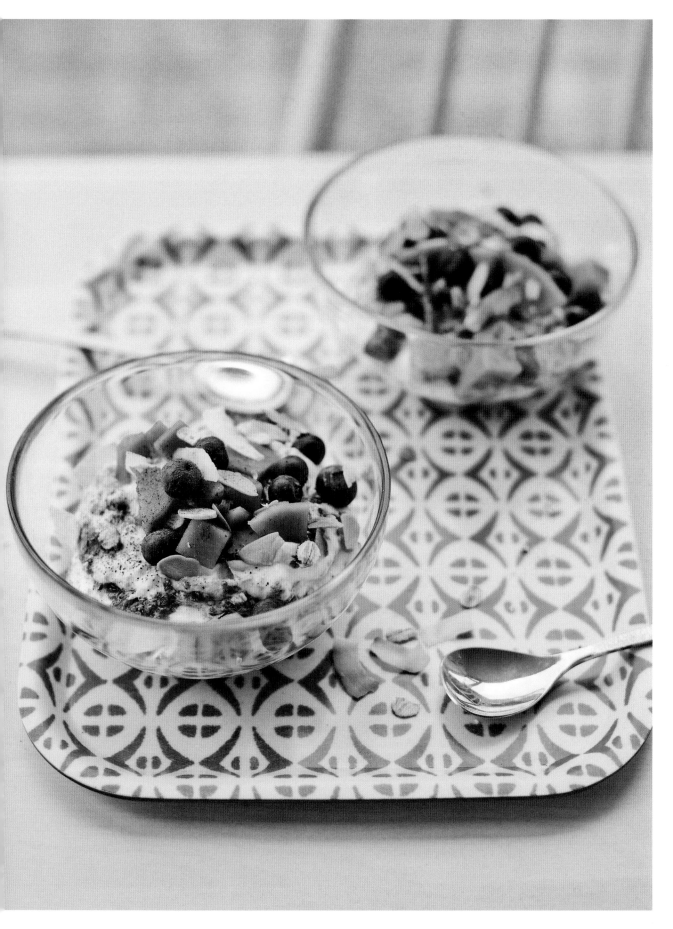

BAKED AVOCADO WITH EGG & TROUT TARTARE

1 portion gives you ▶ FAT **27.1g** (of which SATURATES **6g**) ▶ CARBOHYDRATE **2.8g** (of which SUGARS **1.4g**) ▶ FIBRE **3.8g** ▶ PROTEIN **17.1g** ▶ SALT **1.6g**

Like a kangaroo with a little one in its pouch, in this breakfast the avocado cradles all the other ingredients in its hollow. The smooth texture of the avocado along with the trout, lime, chives and eggs blend deliciously into a warm velvety mélange. If you like the idea of luxuriating in a comforting and indulgent recipe first thing in the morning, secure in the knowledge that it ticks all the nutritional boxes, then this is for you: avocado (good fats), egg and trout (protein) and veggies (carbs). The scooped-out avocado yields enough space for the egg and you can use any leftover avocado scoopings in the tartare. Perfect, and super-simple!

SERVES **2**

PREP TIME: **10 minutes**

COOKING TIME: **25 minutes**

1 large avocado

2 free-range, organic eggs

pinch of dried chilli flakes

TROUT TARTARE

55g (2oz) smoked trout, cut into small pieces

4 radishes, diced

2.5cm (1in) piece of cucumber, quartered, deseeded and diced

1 tbsp snipped chives

juice of 1 lime

Heat the oven to 180°C/350°F/Gas Mark 4.

Start by halving the avocado and taking out the stone. I stick my knife into the stone, twist it, and it comes out pretty easily. Scoop out some of the avocado flesh with a spoon to make room for the egg and save it to use later. Place the avocado halves in a small baking tray, cut-side up, and scrunch up some foil around them to keep the avocados upright and stable.

Crack an egg into a small jug, then pour it into the hollow in one of the avocado halves. Repeat with the second egg and avocado half. Pop the avocados into the oven and cook for 20–25 minutes until the egg white is cooked but the yolks remain slightly runny.

While they are cooking, make the trout tartare. Gently mix together all the ingredients in a bowl.

Place the baked avocados on serving plates and spoon the trout tartare on top. Sprinkle the chilli flakes over and enjoy.

GF DF V

TOFU & SPRING ONION PANCAKES

1 portion gives you ▸ FAT **14.8g** (of which SATURATES **2.8g**) ▸ CARBOHYDRATE **8g** (of which SUGARS **6.8g**) ▸ FIBRE **3.4g** ▸ PROTEIN **15.1g** ▸ SALT **0.85g**

Pancakes in the morning conjure up reminiscences of stacked-up breakfasts in America – such a delicious thought. These pancakes are savoury, and come with a double dose of protein thanks to the addition of tofu. You can find silken tofu in small cartons in the ethnic food sections of your local supermarkets, or in health food shops or Asian grocers – it's an ambient product (on the shelves), rather than chilled. The unusual flavours in this dish add a bit of excitement to any brekkie session. As we know, variety is the spice of life.

SERVES **2**

PREP TIME: **20 minutes**

COOKING TIME: **8 minutes**

140g (5oz) silken tofu, drained well

2 free-range, organic eggs

½ tsp ground turmeric

4 spring onions, finely chopped

2 tbsp chopped coriander leaves

cold-pressed rapeseed oil, for frying

pink or sea salt and cracked black pepper

2 handfuls of rocket leaves, to serve

FRESH TOMATO SAUCE

3 good-size, vine-ripened tomatoes, diced

2cm (¾in) piece of fresh root ginger, peeled and grated

2 tbsp chopped coriander leaves

1 medium-hot green chilli, deseeded and diced

juice of ½–1 lime

Mash the tofu in a bowl with the back of a fork until almost smooth.

Lightly beat the eggs in a separate mixing bowl and stir in the mashed tofu, turmeric, spring onions and coriander. Season with salt and pepper and set aside while you make the fresh tomato sauce.

Put the tomatoes in a bowl. Squeeze the ginger through your fingers to extract the juice – you can do this over the bowl of tomatoes – then stir in the coriander, chilli and lime juice to taste. Discard the ginger flesh. Season the mixture with salt and pepper and set aside while you cook the pancakes.

Heat a splash of oil in a large frying pan over a medium heat. Spoon about 50ml (2fl oz) of the tofu mixture per pancake into the pan and cook three at a time for 2 minutes on each side, or until set and light golden. Drain on kitchen paper and keep the cooked pancakes warm in a low oven while you make three more pancakes (the batter makes about six in total).

Serve the pancakes with a good spoonful of the tomato sauce by the side and a handful of rocket leaves.

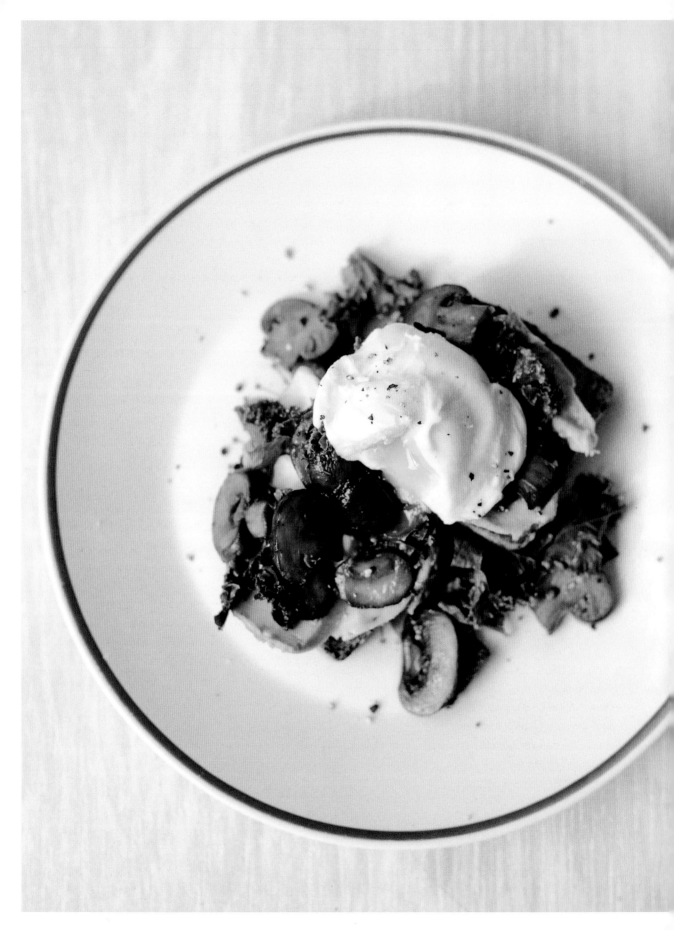

(V)

EGGS FROM THE 'FOREST'

1 portion gives you ▶ FAT **26.5g** (of which SATURATES **5.4g**) ▶ CARBOHYDRATE **30.2g** (of which SUGARS **2.7g**) ▶ FIBRE **5.2g** ▶ PROTEIN **15.8g** ▶ SALT **0.8g**

I couldn't legitimately claim to call my blog *Fitness On Toast* if I didn't whip up the occasional recipe on toast! This doorstep-thick slice of toasted soda bread is towering with goodness. Foraging has forever been part of Scandinavian culinary heritage (popularised more recently by the likes of the restaurant Noma reaching the status of 'best restaurant in the world') and this breakfast plays on that trend. I recommend sprinkling truffle-infused oil on top of the eggs to make your breakfast feel a little extra luxuriant, extra delicious and more genuinely foraged!

SERVES **2**

PREP TIME: **20 minutes**

COOKING TIME: **10 minutes**

1–2 tbsp cold-pressed rapeseed oil

200g (7oz) chestnut mushrooms (or you could use a mixture of different types), sliced

85g (3oz) kale or spinach, tough stalks removed and leaves roughly chopped

1 tsp fresh lemon thyme or regular thyme, plus extra to serve

1 garlic clove, finely chopped (optional)

1 medium-hot red chilli, deseeded and chopped, or a large pinch of dried chilli flakes (optional)

2 slices Spelt & Quinoa Soda Bread (see p.129), or bread of choice

1 small avocado, cut in half, stone removed, mashed or sliced

squeeze of lemon juice

2 large free-range, organic eggs

pink or sea salt and cracked black pepper

Start by heating a small saucepan of water until it almost comes to the boil. This is ready to poach the eggs.

At the same time, heat the oil in a large frying pan and fry the mushrooms for 5 minutes or until they start to turn golden.

Add the kale, thyme, garlic and chilli, if using, and cook for another minute until the kale starts to soften – you don't want it to lose its vibrant colour.

Break the eggs, one at a time, into a small cup. Swirl the simmering water in the pan, add the eggs and reduce the heat to low. Poach the eggs for 3 minutes or until the whites are set but the yolks remain runny.

Toast the bread.

You're now ready to serve – layer the ingredients on top of the toast, starting with the avocado and then the mushroom mixture. Add a squeeze of lemon juice and top each serving with a poached egg. Season with salt and pepper to taste and serve with extra thyme.

GF V

SOUFFLÉ OMELETTE WITH ASPARAGUS & WALNUTS

1 portion gives you ▶ FAT **24g** (of which SATURATES **7.6g**) ▶ CARBOHYDRATE **1.8g** (of which SUGARS **1.5g**) ▶ FIBRE **1.5g** ▶ PROTEIN **12.8g** ▶ SALT **1g**

One of my all-time favourite ways to start the day is with an omelette. This version is light and fluffy as a cloud, and with the velvety smoothness of the goat's cheese is truly melt-in-your-mouth divine!

SERVES **1–2**

PREP TIME: **10 minutes**

COOKING TIME: **10 minutes**

85g (3oz) asparagus spears, ends snapped off

extra virgin olive oil, for cooking and drizzling

15g (½oz) walnut halves

50g (1¾oz) baby spinach leaves

½ tsp finely chopped rosemary (optional)

2 free-range, organic eggs, separated

10g (¼oz) unsalted butter or coconut oil

20g (¾oz) goat's cheese log, cut into pieces

pink or sea salt and cracked black pepper

Heat a griddle pan over a medium heat and, while it is heating, toss the asparagus in a splash of olive oil. Chargrill the spears for 5–8 minutes, turning occasionally, until just tender and smoky in flavour.

Meanwhile, toast the walnuts in a frying pan for 3 minutes, turning once, until they start to colour. Remove the nuts from the pan and leave to cool slightly before breaking them into small pieces.

Next, add a splash of olive oil to the frying pan, then add the spinach and rosemary, if using, and sauté for a few minutes, turning the leaves now and then so they cook evenly and soften slightly. Remove the leaves from the pan with a slotted spoon and set aside.

Now's the time to make the omelette. Season the egg yolks with salt and pepper and whisk with a fork. Put the egg whites in a large, clean bowl and, using an electric hand whisk, beat until they form soft peaks.

Gently fold the egg yolks into the whites, trying not to lose any of the precious air, until combined.

Melt the butter or coconut oil in the frying pan over a medium-low heat, scrape the fluffy egg mixture into the pan and spread it out in an even layer with a spatula. Cook the omelette for 2–3 minutes until the base is light golden – turn the heat down slightly if it browns too quickly. Once golden, use the spatula to carefully turn the omelette over and cook the other side for a couple of minutes until just set.

Just before the omelette is ready, place the spinach and goat's cheese on top to warm through and allow the cheese to melt slightly. Transfer the omelette to a plate and top with the asparagus. Scatter over the walnuts before serving. If you're feeling hungry, eat the whole thing, otherwise cut it in half to serve two people.

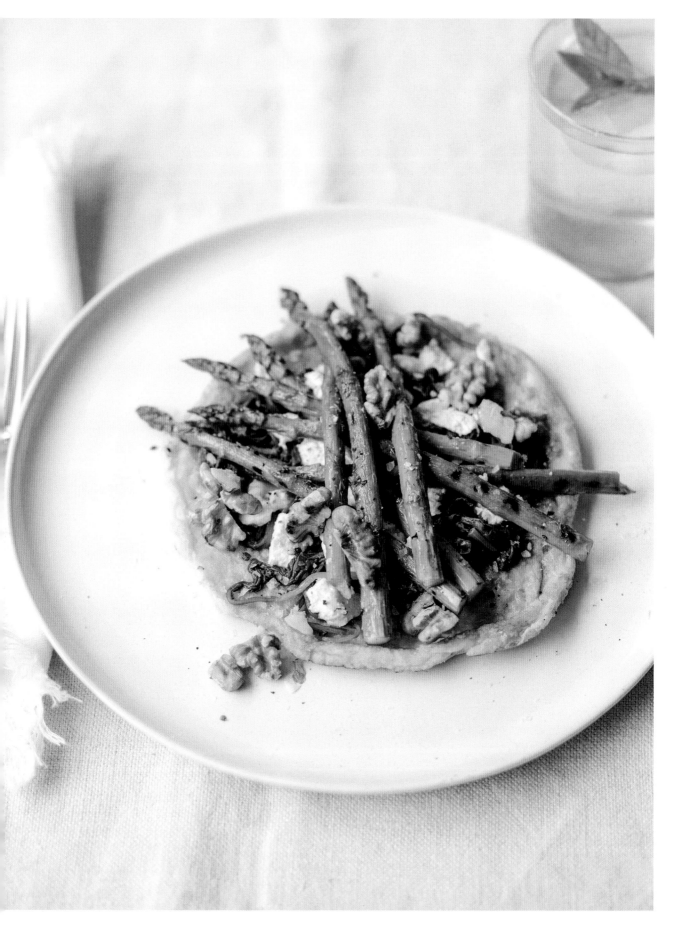

LUNCHES

One of the keys to maintaining a healthy diet is to stay a step ahead, and you can do this by planning your lunch the day before. A degree of simple organisation will help you to ensure that whatever your day throws at you, you're all set! The lunches in this section are perfect for an on-the-go lifestyle and plenty can be popped into a container and taken to the office. Many can be whipped up by simply raiding the fridge and the store cupboard – they rely on simple, fresh ingredients. They're all super-healthy and designed to be filling; you can have confidence that you're nourishing your body with delicious food, to keep yourself going right through to dinner time.

ASIAN BROTH WITH CHICKEN & MINT

1 portion gives you ▶ FAT **9.9g** (of which SATURATES **3.5g**) ▶ CARBOHYDRATE **36.8g** (of which SUGARS **12.5g**)
▶ FIBRE **7.8g** ▶ PROTEIN **42.5g** ▶ SALT **0.9g**

The longer you leave the spices to infuse in this broth, the more intense the flavour will grow; it's as if there's no end in sight to the flavour force! If you choose to take it with you to work, it's worth constructing it in situ. Keep the spiced stock hot in a flask (or heat it once at work) and pour it over the chicken, veg and cooked noodles, then sprinkle with the mint, beansprouts and chilli.

SERVES **2**

PREP TIME: **15 minutes, plus infusing**

COOKING TIME: **20 minutes**

800ml (1⅓ pints) good-quality, low-salt chicken stock

5 cardamom pods, split

3 star anise

1 thumb-sized piece of fresh root ginger, sliced into rounds

250g (9oz) sweet potato, peeled and cut into julienne strips, or 140g (5oz) brown rice noodles

2 large spring onions, sliced diagonally, white and green parts separated

1 handful of long-stem broccoli, trimmed

2 cooked skinless, boneless chicken breasts, shredded into strips

1 good handful of sugar snap peas, sliced diagonally

leaves from 2 mint sprigs

½ medium-hot red chilli, deseeded and diced

1 handful of beansprouts

cracked black pepper

Pour the stock into a saucepan and add the cardamom, star anise and ginger. Bring the stock almost to the boil, then turn the heat down to low, cover with the lid, and simmer for 15 minutes. Turn off the heat and leave the stock to steep for at least 15 minutes, or longer if you have time (overnight is good).

When you're ready to make the soup, scoop out the flavourings and discard them. Reheat the stock to simmering point and add the sweet potato 'noodles', if using. (If opting for the brown rice noodles, cook them separately following the pack instructions, then drain and refresh under cold running water. Add them to the broth just before serving to heat through.)

Add the white part of the spring onions and the broccoli florets to the stock at the same time as the sweet potato 'noodles' and simmer for 2–3 minutes until the vegetables are just tender. Season with pepper, stir in the chicken, sugar snap peas and half of the mint for the last minute of cooking.

Ladle the soup into large, shallow bowls and scatter over the remaining mint, chilli and the beansprouts as you serve.

COCONUT, LENTIL & CARDAMOM SOUP

1 portion gives you ▸ FAT **7.2g** (of which SATURATES **5g**) ▸ CARBOHYDRATE **40.3g** (of which SUGARS **11.7g**) ▸ FIBRE **4.9g** ▸ PROTEIN **12.9g** ▸ SALT **0.4g**

This is a homely, warming and filling bowl of comfort with spices that are great for boosting digestive health. I like to add spinach leaves at the end and just let them wilt so that they retain their nutrients.

SERVES **4**

PREP TIME: **20 minutes**

COOKING TIME: **35 minutes**

1 tbsp coconut oil

1 large onion, chopped

3 carrots, quartered lengthways and sliced

1 large celery stick, thinly sliced

1 thumb-sized piece of fresh root ginger, peeled and grated

2 garlic cloves, chopped

2 bay leaves

2 tsp garam masala

4 cardamom pods, split

1 tsp ground turmeric

175g (6oz) red split lentils

500ml (18fl oz) good-quality, low-salt vegetable stock

500ml (18fl oz) unsweetened coconut drinking milk

a few handfuls of baby spinach leaves (optional)

a squeeze of lime

cracked black pepper

ROASTED BEETROOT RAITA (optional)

1 roast beetroot, peeled and diced

6 tbsp thick plain live yogurt or dairy-free alternative

1 tsp nigella seeds

Heat the oil in a large saucepan and fry the onion for 5 minutes, stirring often, until softened. Next, add the carrots, celery, ginger, garlic, bay leaves, spices and lentils and cook for a couple of minutes, stirring.

Pour in the stock and coconut milk and bring to the boil, then turn the heat down to medium-low and simmer, part-covered with the lid, for 25 minutes, or until the lentils are tender and turning mushy.

You can serve the soup chunky at this point. Alternatively, if you want to serve it puréed, pick out the bay leaves and cardamom – these are quite easy to find as they rise to the top. Season with pepper and, if you like, stir in a few handfuls of spinach and let them cook in the heat of the soup, then purée until thick and smooth.

If serving the soup topped with the beetroot raita – it adds a wonderful colour contrast – mix all the ingredients together and place a large spoonful on top of the soup, then finish with a good squeeze of lime and a grinding of black pepper.

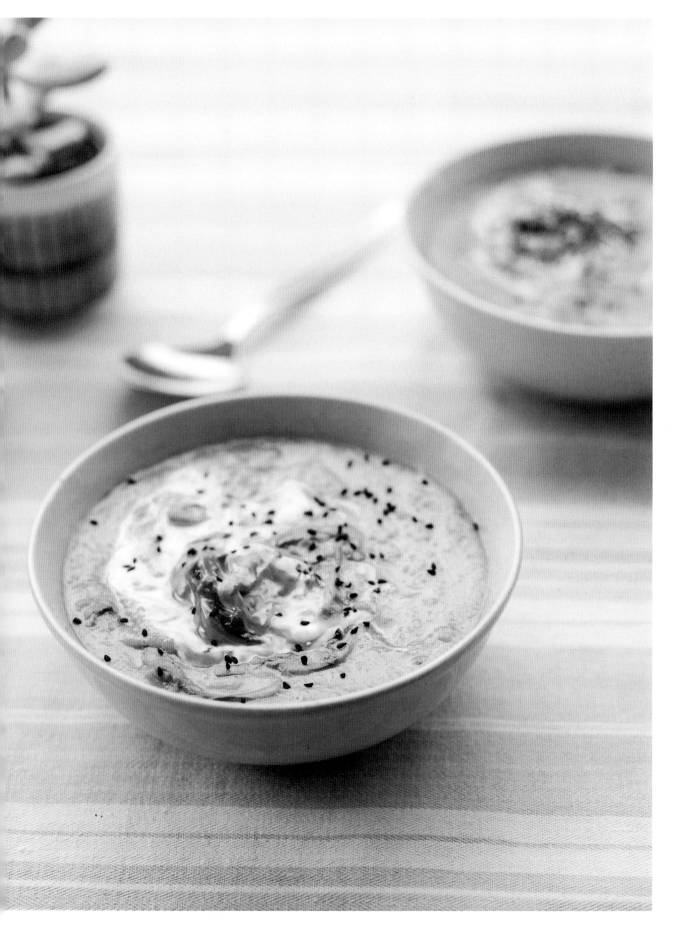

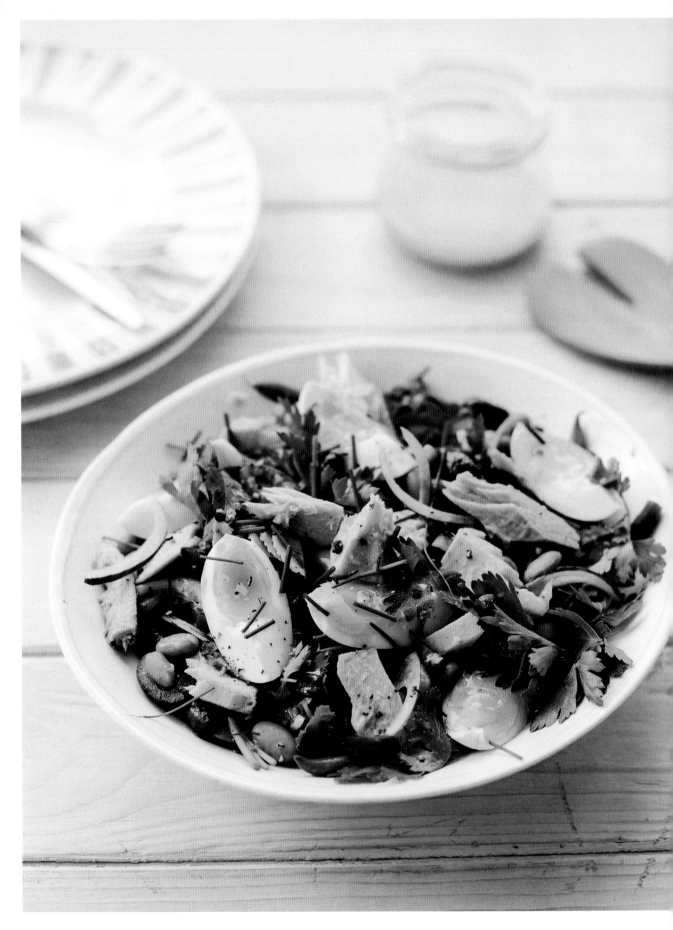

TUNA, EDAMAME & CAPER SALAD WITH MUSTARD DRESSING

1 portion gives you ▶ FAT 22.2g (of which SATURATES 4.7g) ▶ CARBOHYDRATE 20.4g (of which SUGARS 3.4g) ▶ FIBRE 10g ▶ PROTEIN 38.4g ▶ SALT 2g

I love this reinvention of a classic tuna salad. High in protein and low in calories, it is remarkable!

SERVES **2**

PREP TIME: **20 minutes**

50g (1¾oz) fine green beans, halved

50g (1¾oz) frozen edamame beans, defrosted

400g (14oz) can mixed beans, drained and rinsed

1 celery stick, finely sliced

¼ small red onion, finely sliced (optional)

10 pitted kalamata olives, halved

1 tbsp capers, drained

2 handfuls of flatleaf parsley leaves, torn

2 tbsp snipped chives (use the flowers if you have them, too)

115g (4oz) can tuna in spring water, flaked

2 hard-boiled free-range, organic eggs, peeled and quartered

pink or sea salt and cracked black pepper

MUSTARD DRESSING

4 tsp extra virgin olive oil

juice of 1 large lemon

1 tsp Dijon mustard

1 small garlic clove, peeled

First steam the green beans until just tender, then cool them under cold running water to stop them cooking any further.

While the beans are cooking, put the ingredients for the dressing in a small jar, cover with the lid and shake well until combined. Season with salt and pepper and set aside.

To assemble the salad, I like to arrange it in layers in jars to take to work, but you could serve it in a big bowl as described here. Lightly toss together the green beans, edamame, mixed beans, celery, red onion, if using, olives, capers, parsley and half of the chives in a large, shallow serving bowl.

Pour half of the dressing over the bean mixture and lightly toss until combined. Top with the tuna and hard-boiled eggs and finish with a sprinkling of the remaining chives. Taste and pour over more of the dressing if you think it's needed.

SIMPLE SALAD WITH CRAYFISH & CITRUS DRESSING

1 portion gives you ▶ FAT **19.9g** (of which SATURATES **3.6g**) ▶ CARBOHYDRATE **15.8g** (of which SUGARS **5.4g**) ▶ FIBRE **7.5g** ▶ PROTEIN **23.6g** ▶ SALT **0.9g**

We Swedes are fixated on crayfish, and we celebrate its deliciousness with an annual party, in August, called *Kräftskiva* – an elaborate excuse for the country to indulge in snaps, song and shellfish!

SERVES **2**

PREP TIME: **15 minutes**

COOKING TIME: **5 minutes**

200g (7oz) broad beans, shelled, or 100g (3½oz) canned flageolet beans, drained and rinsed

1 tbsp pumpkin seeds

100g (3½oz) mixed watercress, spinach and rocket salad

2 handfuls of sugar snap peas, sliced diagonally

5cm (2in) piece of cucumber, sliced into ribbons using a vegetable peeler, seeds discarded

1 small avocado, halved, stone removed, peeled and sliced

1 tbsp snipped chives

175g (6oz) shelled crayfish tails

1 handful of alfalfa sprouts (optional)

pink or sea salt and cracked black pepper

CITRUS DRESSING

4 tbsp freshly squeezed pink grapefruit juice

juice of ½ lemon

1 tbsp extra virgin olive oil

Steam or boil the broad beans for 3 minutes, or until tender. Place the beans under cold running water to cool and pop them out of their grey outer shell to reveal a bright green bean inside. (Alternatively, you could use canned flageolet beans, which just need draining and rinsing.)

Toast the pumpkin seeds in a dry frying pan for a couple of minutes, tossing them, until they start to colour – take care as they can pop.

Put all the ingredients for the dressing in a small jar, cover with the lid and shake well until combined. Season with salt and pepper and set aside.

Put the salad leaves on a serving plate and top with the cooked broad beans, sugar snap peas, cucumber and avocado. Pour three-quarters of the dressing over and toss gently until combined.

Top the salad with the chives and crayfish, and the alfalfa sprouts, if using. Spoon over more of the dressing, if you think it's needed, and scatter the pumpkin seeds over the top just before serving.

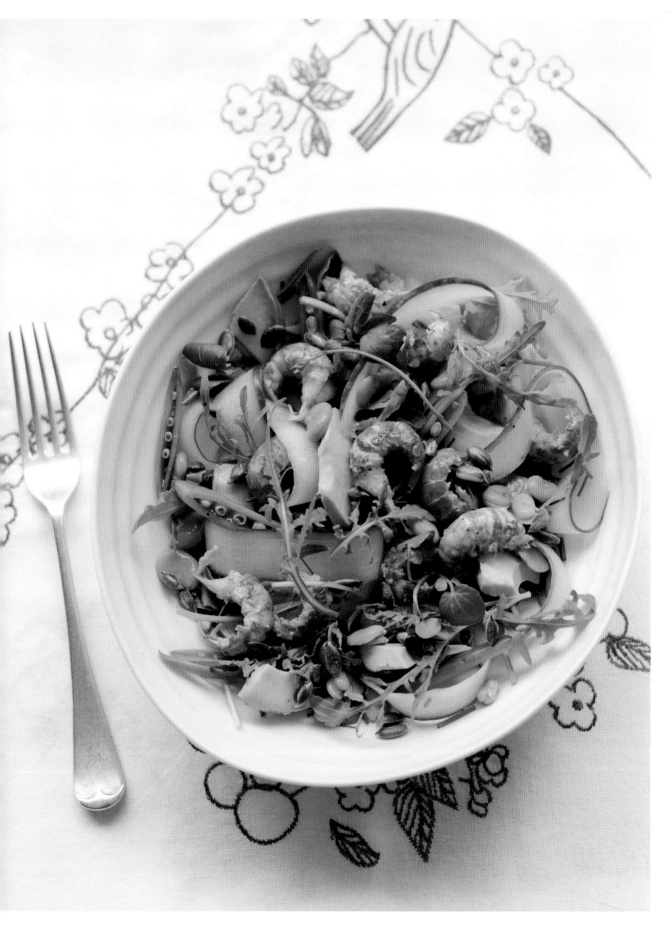

GF **V**

SPICED LENTIL & ARTICHOKE SALAD

1 portion gives you ▶ FAT **13.1g** (of which SATURATES **4.1g**) ▶ CARBOHYDRATE **20g** (of which SUGARS **4.9g**)
▶ FIBRE **7.3g** ▶ PROTEIN **14.7g** ▶ SALT **1.3g**

This Moroccan-style salad bursts with fresh vegetables, rich spices and refreshing fruits, melded to create a debauched orgy of flavours. The lentils are there to provide not just texture, but a great source of plant protein, too.

SERVES **2**

PREP TIME: **20 minutes**

2 large handfuls of rocket leaves

400g (14oz) can green lentils,
   drained

2 cauliflower florets, grated

2 spring onions, finely chopped

5 cherry tomatoes, diced

1 handful of chopped parsley
   leaves

1 handful of chopped coriander
   leaves

½ medium-hot red chilli, deseeded
   and finely chopped

100g (3½oz) grilled artichoke hearts

40g (1½oz) soft goat's cheese or
   feta, crumbled

pink or sea salt and cracked black
   pepper

sprinkling of Za'atar (see p.123)
   (optional)

ORANGE & POMEGRANATE DRESSING

juice and finely grated zest
   of ½ orange

1 tbsp extra virgin olive oil

½ tsp pomegranate molasses

¼ tsp dried chilli flakes

Start by making the dressing. Put everything in a small jar, cover with the lid and shake well until combined. Season the dressing with salt and pepper and set aside.

To make the salad, divide the rocket between two bowls or jars. Mix together the lentils, cauliflower, spring onions, tomatoes, herbs and chilli. Pour the dressing over the top and lightly toss until combined. Spoon on top of the rocket leaves.

Top the salad with the artichokes and goat's cheese and serve sprinkled with a little za'atar, if you like.

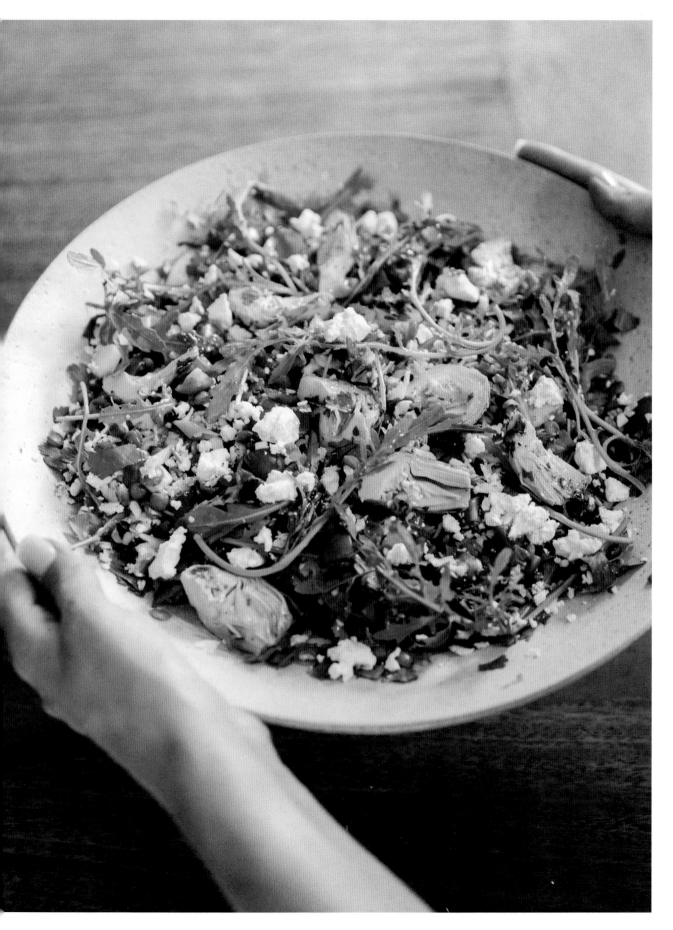

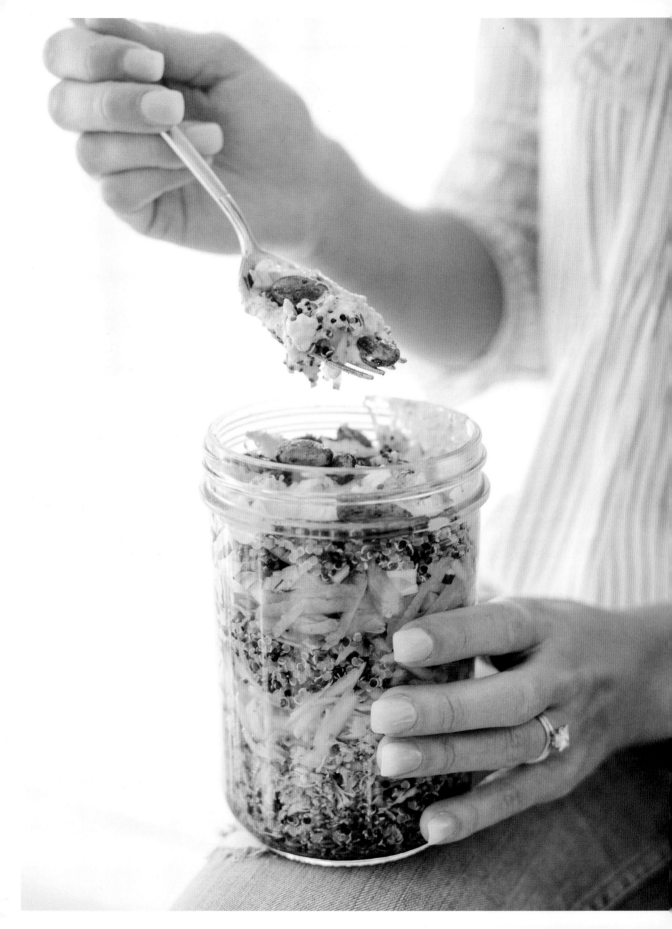

RAINBOW SALAD WITH ROASTED SPICED ALMONDS

1 portion gives you ▸ FAT 25.5g (of which SATURATES 2.9g) ▸ CARBOHYDRATE 32.2g (of which SUGARS 7g) ▸ FIBRE 4.6g ▸ PROTEIN 14.4g ▸ SALT 1.8g

Certain grains and seeds are incredibly rich in vegetable protein – quinoa is chief among them. This salad works beautifully to take to work, layered up in rainbow colours in a jar.

SERVES **2**

PREP TIME: **20 minutes**

COOKING TIME: **15 minutes**

60g (2¼oz) mixed black, red and white quinoa

½ tsp ground turmeric

½ tsp vegetable bouillon powder

2 broccoli florets, coarsely grated (use the stalks, too)

1 yellow courgette, coarsely grated

1 carrot, coarsely grated

½ small red onion, diced (optional)

1 large handful of basil leaves, roughly torn

1 large handful of parsley leaves, chopped

2 tbsp houmous

Roasted Spiced Almonds (see p.122)

pink or sea salt and cracked black pepper

LEMON & CUMIN DRESSING

2 tbsp extra virgin olive oil

finely grated zest of 1 unwaxed lemon

juice of ½ lemon

¼ tsp cumin seeds

Pour the quinoa into a saucepan, cover with water and bring to the boil. Stir in the turmeric and bouillon powder, turn the heat to low and cover the pan with the lid. Simmer for 15 minutes, or until tender – the quinoa should still retain a little crunch. Drain the quinoa and tip it into a serving bowl.

While the quinoa is cooking, put all the ingredients for the dressing in a small jar, cover with the lid and shake well until combined. Season with salt and pepper and set aside.

This colourful salad looks great arranged in layers in a jar (it makes enough for 2 decent-sized jars), so starting from the bottom, pour in some of the dressing then top with a layer of quinoa, broccoli and courgette, then a second layer of quinoa. Follow this with a layer of carrot, onion, if using, the herbs and the remaining quinoa. Pour over the remaining dressing.

Top with houmous and roasted spiced nuts – if not eating the salad straight away, take these to work separately in pots. The salad tastes best served at room temperature.

(V)

BROAD BEAN, MINT & RICOTTA SMÖRGÅS

1 portion gives you ▶ FAT 13.9g (of which SATURATES 4.1g) ▶ CARBOHYDRATE 38.9g (of which SUGARS 3.8g) ▶ FIBRE 7.3g ▶ PROTEIN 16.9g ▶ SALT 1.3g

Like the Brits, we Swedes take our sandwiches very seriously, as they fall under the umbrella of the sacred pastime *fika* (see p.38). Here, the pretty pale green toppings are scrumptious – be warned this sandwich is incredibly moreish! For some extra topping flare, I'd suggest adding thin slices of beef or lamb, hard-boiled egg, or (my favourite) smoked salmon!

SERVES **2**

PREP TIME: **15 minutes**

COOKING TIME: **10 minutes**

200g (7oz) shelled broad beans (or you could use fresh or frozen peas)

85g (3oz) ricotta cheese

15g (½oz) mint leaves, roughly chopped, plus extra to serve

1 handful of basil leaves

juice and finely grated zest of 1 unwaxed lemon

GARLIC TOASTS

4 small or 2 large, thick slices sourdough bread, or bread of choice

1 garlic clove, peeled and halved

extra virgin olive oil, avocado oil or hemp seed oil, for drizzling

pink or sea salt and cracked black pepper

radish sprouts, to garnish (optional)

EXTRA TOPPINGS IDEAS

- Scrambled egg with diced green chilli, smoked paprika, spring onions and diced red pepper
- Marinated salmon with fennel (see p.82)
- Mashed soft-boiled egg with chopped dill, capers, celery, crème fraîche and Dijon mustard
- Crumbled soft goat's cheese, sliced black figs, a drizzle of good-quality raw honey and toasted chopped walnuts
- Mashed avocado, cooked garlic, prawns, lime juice, diced red onion, broccoli sprouts, toasted black sesame seeds and drizzle of extra virgin oil or avocado oil

Steam the broad beans or boil them in a small amount of water until tender. Drain the beans, if necessary, and cool them under cold running water. I like to pop the beans out of their tough grey outer shell to reveal a bright green bean inside.

Put the beans in a blender with the ricotta, mint, basil and lemon juice and zest. Season with salt and pepper and blend until smooth and creamy. Add a splash of water if the mixture is too thick – you want it to be a thick, spreadable consistency. Taste and add more salt and pepper, if needed, then set aside.

To make the garlic toasts, put the bread on a griddle pan over a medium-high heat and toast on each side until crisp and golden. Rub each slice with the cut side of the garlic and drizzle over a little oil. Cut the toasts in half and top with a thick layer of the broad bean mixture.

Before serving, drizzle with a little extra oil and scatter over some radish sprouts, if you like, and extra mint leaves. The toasts are delicious served simply, or you could add an extra topping from the list of suggestions here.

GF DF V

ROASTED AUBERGINE & SUNDRIED TOMATO SALAD

1 portion gives you ▶ FAT **31.5g** (of which SATURATES **3.6g**) ▶ CARBOHYDRATE **10.2g** (of which SUGARS **8.4g**)
▶ FIBRE **5.2g** ▶ PROTEIN **5.3g** ▶ SALT **0.8g**

This is a hugely adaptable recipe. You can eat it on its own, as a salad as part of a mezze, in a wrap, on toasted bread, as a salsa with fish or meat, or with beans make it more substantial and serve with bulgur wheat and a sprinkling of toasted pine nuts. However you serve it, it represents a delectable burst of flavour to electrify any dish!

SERVES **2**

PREP TIME: **15 minutes**

COOKING TIME: **30 minutes**

1 aubergine

½ red pepper, deseeded and diced

2 sundried tomatoes in oil, finely
chopped, plus 1 tbsp oil
from the jar

1 tomato, diced

1 small garlic clove, finely chopped
(optional)

1 tbsp diced red onion

2 large handfuls of parsley, leaves
finely chopped

¼ tsp dried chilli flakes

1 tbsp extra virgin olive oil

juice of ½ lemon

pink or sea salt and cracked black
pepper

2 tbsp toasted pine nuts, to garnish

Heat the oven to 220°C/425°F/Gas Mark 7. Put the aubergine on a baking tray and roast for 30 minutes or until the inside is meltingly soft. Leave to cool slightly, then slice it in half lengthways and scoop out the flesh, discarding any overly seedy bits as well as the skin.

Finely chop the aubergine flesh and place it in a bowl with the red pepper, the sundried and fresh tomatoes, the garlic, if using, onion, parsley and chilli flakes.

Mix together the oil from the sundried tomatoes with the extra virgin olive oil and lemon juice. Season with salt and pepper. Pour the dressing over the aubergine salad and scatter the pine nuts over the top before serving the salad slightly warm or at room temperature.

BAKED SWEET POTATO WITH CURRIED APPLE SLAW

1 portion gives you ▶ FAT **23.2g** (of which SATURATES **4.4g**) ▶ CARBOHYDRATE **63.8g** (of which SUGARS **27.2g**)
▶ FIBRE **11.4g** ▶ PROTEIN **14.7g** ▶ SALT **0.9g**

Sweet potato is one of those rare and beautiful things of nature: healthy, yet utterly scrumptious.
For a non-veggie option, I like to top this dish with flakes of either smoked mackerel or trout, too.

SERVES **2**

PREP TIME: **15 minutes**

COOKING TIME: **1 hour**

2 sweet potatoes, about 200g (7oz)
  each
2 tbsp cashew nuts
1 heaped tbsp pumpkin seeds
splash of extra virgin olive oil,
  pumpkin oil or avocado oil, for
  drizzling
pink or sea salt and cracked black
  pepper

CURRIED APPLE SLAW
1 small green eating apple, cored
  and coarsely grated
juice of ½ lemon, plus an extra
  squeeze
100g (3½oz) red cabbage,
  shredded
1 carrot, coarsely grated
1 small turnip, peeled and coarsely
  grated
1 tbsp shelled hemp seeds
  (optional)
6 tbsp plain live yogurt or dairy-free
  alternative
½–1 tsp medium curry powder
¼ tsp ground turmeric
3 tbsp snipped chives

Heat the oven to 200°C/400°F/Gas Mark 6. Bake the sweet potatoes for
50 minutes–1 hour until tender.

While the potatoes are cooking, make the slaw. Put the apple in a bowl
and squeeze over a little lemon juice to stop it turning brown. Stir in the
cabbage, carrot, turnip and hemp seeds, if using.

Mix together the yogurt, remaining lemon juice, curry powder and
turmeric in a separate bowl. Season with salt and pepper and pour
the dressing over the slaw. Add the chives and turn until everything
is mixed together. Taste and add more curry powder if you like a spicier
slaw. Set aside until ready to serve.

Toast the cashews in a large, dry frying pan over a medium-low heat,
tossing occasionally, until they start to turn golden and smell toasted –
this takes about 4 minutes. Tip the nuts into a bowl and leave to cool.
Repeat with the pumpkin seeds, toasting them for about 2–3 minutes –
take care as they can pop in the pan.

To serve, make a cut in the top of each baked potato and open out.
Top with a good spoonful of the curried apple slaw and a sprinkling
of nuts and seeds.

MARINATED SALMON WITH FENNEL

1 portion gives you ▶ FAT **29.1g** (of which SATURATES **5.1g**) ▶ CARBOHYDRATE **6.5g** (of which SUGARS **5g**) ▶ FIBRE **6.4g** ▶ PROTEIN **24.5g** ▶ SALT **0.7g**

Perhaps one of my favourite dishes in this book, this marinated salmon is captivatingly stunning to behold, super-fresh to taste, and vibrant to all the senses. It's a real showstopper! Delicate and slender slices of salmon are offset with tangy fennel and smooth avocado – and yet it is also super-easy to make (but don't tell anyone that, insist it was laborious turmoil – your friends will be so overwhelmed by its beauty they won't question you). The perfect summery lunch dish, it works equally well in the frostier months as a light lunchtime option. And because it's a dish that's certain to impress, it also makes the perfect romantic lunch for two.

SERVES **2**

PREP TIME: **20 minutes**

200g (7oz) very fresh, organic
   salmon fillet, pin-boned and
   skinned, rinsed and patted dry
1 fennel bulb, halved crossways
   and cut into thin strips, fronds
   reserved
½ small red onion, diced
4 radishes, thinly sliced into rounds
leaves from 1 mint sprig
½ small avocado, stone removed,
   peeled and sliced
1 handful of broccoli sprouts
extra virgin olive oil, for drizzling
cracked black pepper

SPICED CITRUS MARINADE
juice of 1½ limes
juice of ½ orange
½ medium-hot red chilli, deseeded
   and diced
pink or sea salt

Cut the salmon into 2cm (¾in) even-sized squares or slice into strips, then place in a bowl.

Put all the ingredients for the marinade in a small jar, cover with the lid and shake well until combined. Season with salt and set aside.

Shortly before serving, pour the dressing over the salmon and leave for 7–10 minutes until the fish turns opaque – you don't want to 'cook' the fish in the juice so keep an eye on the time.

Arrange the fennel, onion, radishes, mint and avocado on two plates. Top with the salmon and spoon some of the marinade over each serving. Turn gently until combined, then sprinkle with the fennel fronds and broccoli sprouts. Drizzle over a little olive oil, season with black pepper and serve straight away.

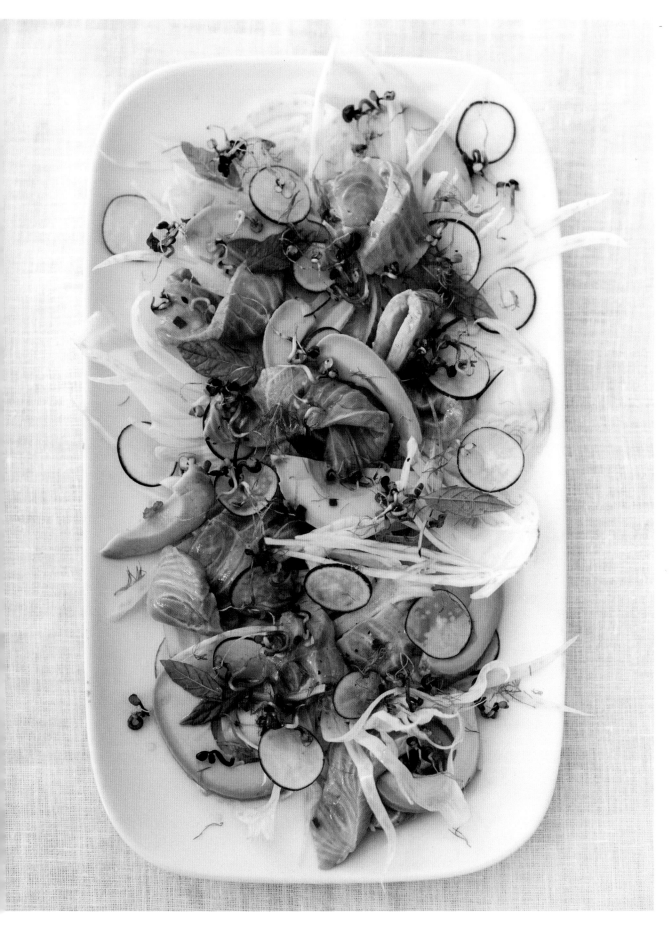

SCANDI SEAWEED WRAPS

Nutritional content will depend upon the filling you choose.

This is my Scandinavian twist on a Japanese-style nori wrap. I use hot horseradish – instead of wasabi – for its potent anti-inflammatory powers. It is also packed with dietary fibre and vitamin C.

SERVES **2**

PREP TIME: **10 minutes, plus pickling**

1 tbsp white wine vinegar

½ tsp good-quality raw honey

¼ tsp sea salt

4cm (1½in) piece of cucumber, sliced

4 nori sheets

1 tbsp Fresh Horseradish Cream
  (see p.93) or ready-made

EXTRA FILLING IDEAS

▶ **Carb:** Cooked quinoa; short-grain brown rice; noodles

▶ **Veg:** Thinly sliced radish, turnip, avocado, spring onion or red onion (left for 10 minutes in hot water); strips of courgette, carrot, red pepper, sugar snaps, celeriac

▶ **Herbs:** Basil; coriander; dill; parsley; chives

▶ **Seeds & sprouts:** Toasted sesame, sunflower or pumpkin seeds; flaxseeds; shelled hemp seeds; alfalfa, broccoli or radish sprouts

▶ **Seafood:** Cooked or smoked salmon; trout; mackerel; prawns; crab; crayfish tails

▶ **Meat:** Cooked chicken, turkey, beef, pork, venison

First make the pickled cucumber. Mix together the vinegar, honey and salt in a bowl until the salt dissolves. Stir in the cucumber then massage it with your fingers until it starts to soften. Leave for about 15 minutes to let the cucumber take on the flavours of the pickle.

Using a pair of tongs, hold a sheet of nori over a hob and toast briefly on both sides – it takes just seconds to crisp up.

Spread a smear of the horseradish cream down one side of each nori sheet and top with your choice of toppings, followed by some of the cucumber pickle. Roll up the nori sheets into a cylinder then slice diagonally in half. Eat straight away – or assemble just before eating to prevent the nori turning soggy.

MINI CHICKPEA BURGERS WITH TAHINI-YOGURT DRIZZLE

1 portion gives you ▶ FAT **19g** (of which SATURATES **3g**) ▶ CARBOHYDRATE **26.1g** (of which SUGARS **6.7g**) ▶ FIBRE **3.4g** ▶ PROTEIN **14.5g** ▶ SALT **0.8g**

These veggie mini-burgers, served in lettuce-leaf 'cups', are perfect for sating the inner caveman!

MAKES **12** (serves 4)

PREP TIME: **15 minutes**, plus chilling

COOKING TIME: **12 minutes**

400g (14oz) can chickpeas, drained, rinsed and patted dry

2 garlic cloves, finely chopped

1 red onion, grated

55g (2oz) sundried tomatoes in oil, drained and finely chopped

½ red pepper, deseeded and chopped

1 medium-hot red chilli, deseeded and diced

1 tsp dried oregano

1 free-range, organic egg, beaten

4 tbsp gram flour, plus extra for coating

cold-pressed rapeseed oil, for frying

pink or sea salt and cracked black pepper

Little Gem lettuce leaves, separated, to serve

TAHINI-YOGURT DRIZZLE

8 tbsp plain live yogurt or dairy-free alternative

2 tbsp tahini

1 small garlic clove, crushed

juice of ½ lemon

Lightly crush the chickpeas in a food processor or using a stick blender – you don't want a smooth paste, but rather a coarse-textured one with chunks of chickpea.

Scrape the chickpeas into a bowl and stir in the garlic, onion, sundried tomatoes, red pepper, chilli, oregano and egg to make a fairly wet paste. Season with salt and pepper and stir in the gram flour to bind the mixture – it will still be quite loose but will firm up when chilled.

Generously cover a plate with gram flour. Form the chickpea mixture into large walnut-sized balls – it makes about 12 in total – and roll each one in the flour until lightly coated. Place on a plate and chill for 30 minutes to firm up.

Meanwhile, mix together all the ingredients for the tahini-yogurt drizzle, season with salt and pepper and set aside.

To cook the mini burgers, heat enough oil to lightly coat the base of a large frying pan. Put half of the burgers in the pan, flatten the tops with a spatula to make a burger shape, and cook for 2–3 minutes on each side until lightly golden. Drain on kitchen paper while you cook the second batch.

To serve, place a mini burger in a Little Gem lettuce leaf and spoon over some of the tahini-yogurt drizzle.

DINNERS

These are some of my favourite nutritious and scrumptious dinners, from quick weeknight suppers to more elaborate recipes perfect for social occasions or weekends, when you've a little more time to luxuriate in the process. In Sweden, we like to eat like a king in the morning, a prince at lunch and a pauper in the evening – so nothing here is too heavy – but that doesn't mean the dishes will leave you hungry. Dinner is a meal to savour, share with friends, and help you unwind after a long day... enjoy it!

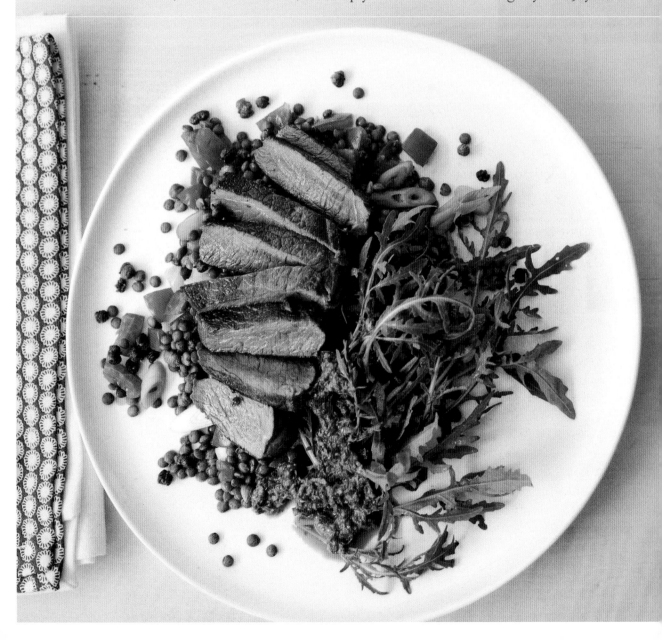

VENISON SALAD WITH FRESH HERB DRESSING

1 portion gives you ▶ FAT **21.6g** (of which SATURATES **3.9g**) ▶ CARBOHYDRATE **10.9g** (of which SUGARS **4g**) ▶ FIBRE **4.3g** ▶ PROTEIN **32.8g** ▶ SALT **1g**

When I was young, my friend's parents would hunt in the forest and I'd walk in to see a deer hanging upside down being prepared for dinner. An excellent source of lean protein, venison packs 50 per cent more protein, kilo for kilo, than the equivalent weight in beef, all for fewer calories! Where possible, opt for wild meat.

SERVES **2**

PREP TIME: **15 minutes**

COOKING TIME: **5 minutes**

250g (9oz) grass-fed venison steak, at room temperature

extra virgin olive oil, for brushing, frying and drizzling

2 tbsp small capers, drained and patted dry

85g (3oz) rocket leaves

100g (3½oz) cooked green or Puy lentils, drained

1 large spring onion, sliced diagonally

3 vine-ripened tomatoes, deseeded and diced

1 tsp balsamic vinegar

pink or sea salt and cracked black pepper

FRESH HERB DRESSING (SERVES 4)

15g (½oz) basil leaves

10g (¼oz) oregano leaves

1 handful of chives

2 tbsp extra virgin olive oil

juice of ½ lemon

1 small garlic clove, peeled and finely chopped

Put the venison in a shallow dish, drizzle over a little oil and season with salt and pepper. Set aside while you make the herb dressing.

Put all the ingredients for the herb dressing in a blender and blitz, adding a splash of water to make a spoonable sauce consistency. Season with salt and pepper and set aside.

Heat a splash of oil in a large frying pan and fry the capers for a minute or two until they turn crisp and golden. Remove from the pan and drain on kitchen paper.

Put the rocket, lentils, spring onion and tomatoes in a shallow serving bowl.

Wipe the frying pan clean, add a splash of oil and heat until almost smoking. Cook the venison for about 2 minutes on each side for rare (3–4 for medium; 4–5 for well-done), then transfer to a board. Cover with foil and leave to rest for 5 minutes.

Thinly slice the venison and place on top of the salad, drizzle over the balsamic vinegar, add a splash of olive oil and top with dollops of the herb dressing.

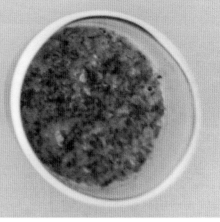

GF DF

MARINATED CHICKEN WITH BUTTERNUT SQUASH & GINGER MASH

1 portion gives you ▶ FAT 17.2g (of which SATURATES 3.9g) ▶ CARBOHYDRATE 25.3g (of which SUGARS 12.4g) ▶ FIBRE 4.1g ▶ PROTEIN 41.7g ▶ SALT 0.9g

A fantastic source of lean protein, no wonder chicken is the staple for a post-workout meal!

SERVES 2

PREP TIME: 20 minutes, plus
  marinating

COOKING TIME: 20 minutes

2 tbsp olive oil

juice of 1 lime

2 tsp mild smoked paprika

1 tsp dried thyme

350g (12oz) skinless, boneless free-
  range mini chicken fillets

pink or sea salt and cracked black
  pepper

steamed long-stem broccoli,
  to serve

BUTTERNUT SQUASH & GINGER MASH

500g (1lb 2oz) squash, peeled,
  deseeded and cut into chunks

2 garlic cloves, peeled and left
  whole

2.5cm (1in) piece of fresh root
  ginger, sliced into rounds

1 medium-hot red chilli, deseeded
  and diced

3–4 tbsp unsweetened coconut
  drinking milk

1 large handful of chopped
  coriander leaves (optional)

Start by making the marinade for the chicken by mixing together the olive oil, lime juice, paprika and thyme in a shallow dish. Season with salt and pepper, add the chicken and turn until it is coated in the marinade. Cover the dish with cling film and leave the chicken to marinate in the fridge for about 1 hour.

Just before you are ready to cook the chicken, make the mash. Put the squash in a saucepan with the garlic and ginger, cover with water and bring to the boil. Turn the heat down, part-cover with the lid, and simmer for 10 minutes or until tender. Drain the pan, pick out the ginger and add the chilli and coconut drinking milk to the squash, then mash until smooth. Season with salt and pepper, and stir in three-quarters of the coriander leaves.

To cook the chicken, heat a griddle pan over a high heat. Remove the chicken from the marinade and chargrill for 5–7 minutes, turning once, or until cooked through – you may need to cook it in two batches. Throw away the marinade.

Reheat the mash if you need to, then spoon it onto two serving plates. Top with the broccoli and chicken and finish off with a sprinkling of the reserved coriander, if you like.

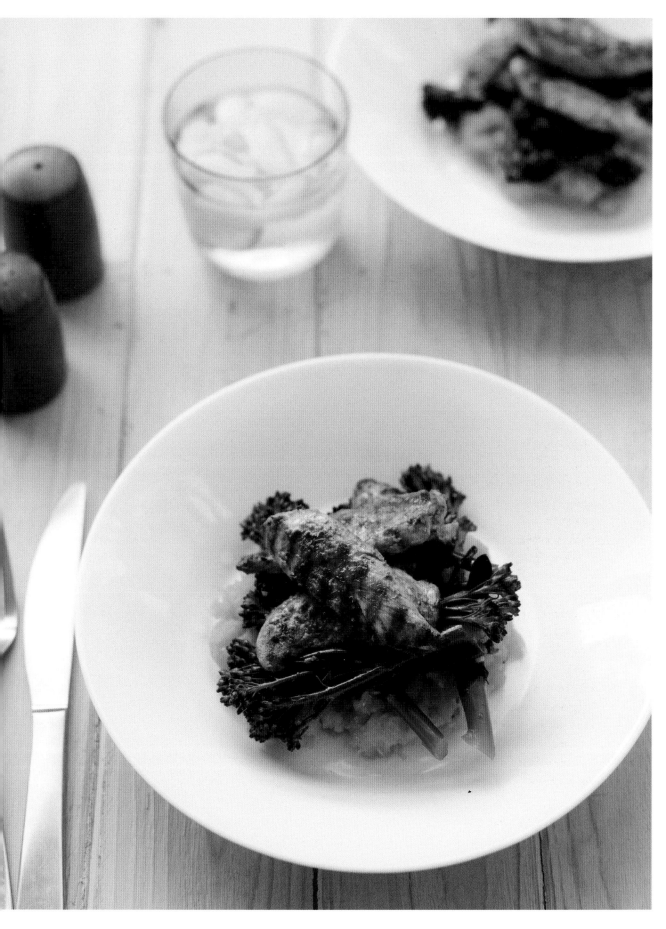

VENISON MEATBALLS WITH BLACKBERRY SAUCE

1 portion gives you ▶ FAT **11.4g** (of which SATURATES **1.8g**) ▶ CARBOHYDRATE **26.1g** (of which SUGARS **11g**) ▶ FIBRE **7.9g** ▶ PROTEIN **33.9g** ▶ SALT **1g**

While you may automatically associate Sweden with meatballs (thanks largely to IKEA and the Swedish Chef from *The Muppet Show*), they're not quite representative of the homemade *köttbullar* we proudly pour our love into! The recipes for *köttbullar* are passed down the maternal lineage, with specific flavour secrets held tightly for generations. Venison is a lean, low-fat red meat that's full of flavour to make great meatballs. These meatballs come with a rich berry sauce and are fantastic served with soft polenta or mashed potato, and steamed hispi cabbage.

SERVES **2**

PREP TIME: **20 minutes, plus chilling**

COOKING TIME: **15 minutes**

70g (2½oz) day-old, gluten-free, seeded bread

275g (9¾oz) venison steaks, minced or very finely chopped

1 small red onion, coarsely grated

½ tsp allspice

cold-pressed rapeseed oil, for frying

1 tbsp chopped dill

pink or sea salt and cracked black pepper

BLACKBERRY SAUCE

200g (7oz) blackberries or blueberries

2 tsp balsamic vinegar

10 juniper berries, crushed

1 tsp good-quality raw honey

½ tsp chia seeds

squeeze of lemon

Blitz the bread in a food processor to make breadcrumbs. Tip the crumbs into a mixing bowl with the venison, onion and allspice, season with salt and pepper and mix everything together with your hands. Shape the venison mixture into 14 walnut-sized balls, then cover with cling film and chill in the refrigerator for 30 minutes to firm up.

Next, make the fruit sauce. Put the blackberries or blueberries in a small saucepan with the vinegar, juniper berries and honey. Bring up to simmering point, then turn the heat down and cook gently for about 5 minutes until reduced and thickened. Press the sauce through a sieve into a bowl and discard any seeds and the juniper berries. Stir the chia seeds into the fruit sauce and add a squeeze of lemon, then set aside to thicken up while you cook the meatballs.

Heat enough oil to coat the base of a large frying pan over a medium heat. Cook the meatballs in two batches for about 5 minutes each, turning them while they cook, until golden all over. Keep the first batch of meatballs warm in a low oven while you cook the second batch.

Serve the meatballs with a good spoonful of the blackberry sauce and steamed hispi cabbage.

TUNA BURGER WITH FRESH PICKLE

1 portion gives you ▶ FAT **19.1g** (of which SATURATES **3.8g**) ▶ CARBOHYDRATE **61g** (of which SUGARS **13.3g**) ▶ FIBRE **3.6g** ▶ PROTEIN **46.5g** ▶ SALT **2g**

Sometimes you just crave a burger, so here's a good recipe to make a super-easy scrumptious dish packed with a high-quality source of protein! This one comes served in a wholegrain bun, spread with tangy lime avocado and topped with a crunchy homemade pickle, but you can garnish it to your taste.

SERVES **2**

PREP TIME: **20 minutes, plus pickling**

COOKING TIME: **5 minutes**

½ avocado, stone removed and
   flesh scooped out

good squeeze of lime juice

2 x 150g (5½oz) sustainably
   sourced, thick tuna steaks

olive oil, for brushing

2 wholegrain buns or bagels, split
   in half and lightly toasted

rocket leaves, to serve

pink or sea salt and cracked black
   pepper

CARROT & RED CABBAGE PICKLE

1 carrot, coarsely grated

85g (3oz) red cabbage, shredded

¼ small red onion, thinly sliced

1cm (½in) piece of fresh root
   ginger, peeled and finely grated

1 tbsp white wine vinegar

1 tsp good-quality raw honey

¼ tsp dried chilli flakes

½ tsp black sesame seeds

To make the carrot and red cabbage pickle, simply mix together all the ingredients in a bowl. Season with salt and pepper and set aside for 30 minutes for the pickle ingredients to meld and mingle.

Mash the avocado with a good squeeze of lime juice, then set aside.

Heat a griddle pan over a high heat. Brush the tuna with a little olive oil, season with salt and pepper and sear for a couple of minutes on each side, or until still slightly pink in the centre.

To assemble the tuna burgers, spoon the avocado over the base of each toasted bun, top with a few rocket leaves, the chargrilled tuna and a good spoonful of the pickle. Finish with the bun lid and serve straight away. You'll need napkins!

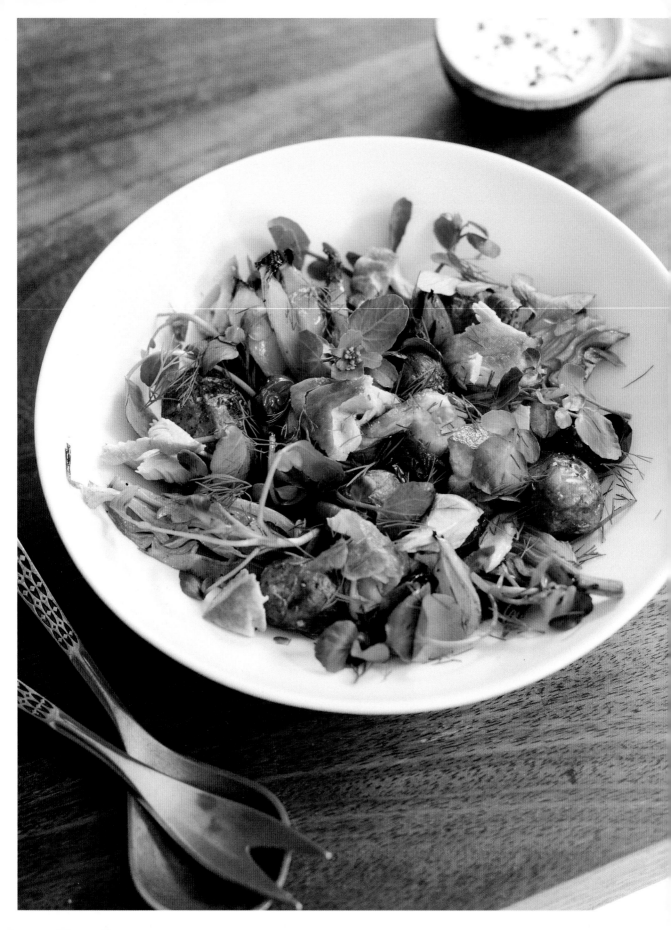

WARM SALAD OF ROASTED SALMON, FENNEL & BABY NEW POTATOES

1 portion gives you ▶ FAT 30g (of which SATURATES 5.7g) ▶ CARBOHYDRATE 44.6g (of which SUGARS 11.9g) ▶ FIBRE 7.9g ▶ PROTEIN 33.5g ▶ SALT 0.7g

This deliciously light meal is cooked in the oven together, meaning you don't have to spin ten plates while trying to orchestrate your evening! Swedes love potatoes and for good reason. With the skins on, they have antioxidant power and provide a slow-releasing energy source.

SERVES **2**

PREP TIME: **20 minutes**

COOKING TIME: **55 minutes**

400g (14oz) baby new potatoes

1½ tbsp extra virgin olive oil, plus extra for drizzling

2 bay leaves

1 onion, cut into wedges

1 fennel bulb, cut into wedges

8 vine-ripened cherry tomatoes

1 handful of lemon thyme sprigs

2 x 150g (5½oz) organic salmon fillets, pin-boned

½ unwaxed lemon, sliced, plus extra wedges, to serve

100g (3½oz) watercress

1 handful of dill, chopped

pink or sea salt and cracked black pepper

FRESH HORSERADISH CREAM (SERVES 4)

1 heaped tbsp fresh horseradish root, peeled and finely grated, or ready-made horseradish sauce

4 tbsp half-fat crème fraîche or cashew cream (see p.94)

1 tbsp white wine vinegar

Heat the oven to 200°C/400°F/Gas Mark 6. Toss the new potatoes in half of the oil, season with salt and pepper, and tip them into a roasting tin. Scrunch the bay leaves in your hand, then place on top of the potatoes and roast for 25 minutes.

Toss the onion, fennel and tomatoes in the remaining oil and add them to the tin with the potatoes. Scatter over the thyme sprigs and return to the oven for a further 20–25 minutes or until everything is cooked through and the potatoes are crisp and golden.

Place the salmon on top of the potatoes and vegetables, drizzle over a little oil, season with salt and pepper and top with a few lemon slices. Return the tin to the oven for a final 10–12 minutes until the salmon is cooked through and lightly coloured.

While the vegetables and salmon are roasting, mix together all the ingredients for the fresh horseradish cream in a small bowl. Alternatively, you can use ready-made horseradish sauce.

To assemble the warm salad, place the watercress on a serving dish, top with the potato and vegetable mixture, discarding the thyme and bay leaves. Flake the salmon on top and drizzle over a little oil, if needed. Serve with a good spoonful of the horseradish sauce and wedges of lemon.

HERRINGS IN OATMEAL WITH RÉMOULADE

1 portion gives you ▶ FAT **39.9g** (of which SATURATES **7.8g**) ▶ CARBOHYDRATE **23.4g** (of which SUGARS **3.8g**) ▶ FIBRE **6.1g** ▶ PROTEIN **37.5g** ▶ SALT **1.3g**

Herring has been a staple of traditional Swedish cuisine since at least the 16th century, and has basically become the idiosyncratic national food, along with meatballs! But while it's typically chopped and marinated, and served cold, this is an altogether understated use of the heroic herring. Filleted herring is pretty economical to buy, quick to cook and full of healthy omega-3 fatty acids. Here, I've coated the fish in a crisp, oatmeal crust, and paired them with a dairy-free rémoulade. Think of them as the deliciously healthy alternative to fish fingers!

SERVES **2**

PREP TIME: **20 minutes, plus soaking**

COOKING TIME: **4 minutes**

4 large or 8 small herring fillets, large bones discarded
English mustard, for brushing
50g (1¾oz) medium oatmeal
1 tbsp ground flaxseeds
cold-pressed rapeseed oil, for frying
mixed leaf salad, to serve

RÉMOULADE

30g (1oz) cashew nuts
85g (3oz) celeriac, peeled and cut into thin matchsticks
juice of 1 small lemon
1 carrot, cut into thin matchsticks
1 tsp Dijon mustard
2 tbsp finely chopped parsley leaves
pink or sea salt and cracked black pepper

To make the rémoulade, soak the cashew nuts in 100ml (3½fl oz) hot water for 1 hour. Tip the nuts and soaking water into a small blender and blend until smooth and creamy. Prepare the celeriac and immediately toss it in the lemon juice to stop it discolouring. Place in a bowl with the carrot and mustard. Pour over the cashew cream, season with salt and pepper and stir until combined. Set aside.

Rinse and pat dry the herring fillets. Spread the English mustard over both sides of each fillet, mix together the oatmeal and flaxseeds, then dunk the fillets in the oatmeal mixture until evenly coated.

Heat enough oil to coat the base of a large frying pan over a medium heat and fry the herring fillets for 2 minutes on each side until crisp and golden.

Divide the rémoulade between two serving plates, sprinkle with parsley, place the crispy herring fillets by the side and serve with a mixed leaf salad.

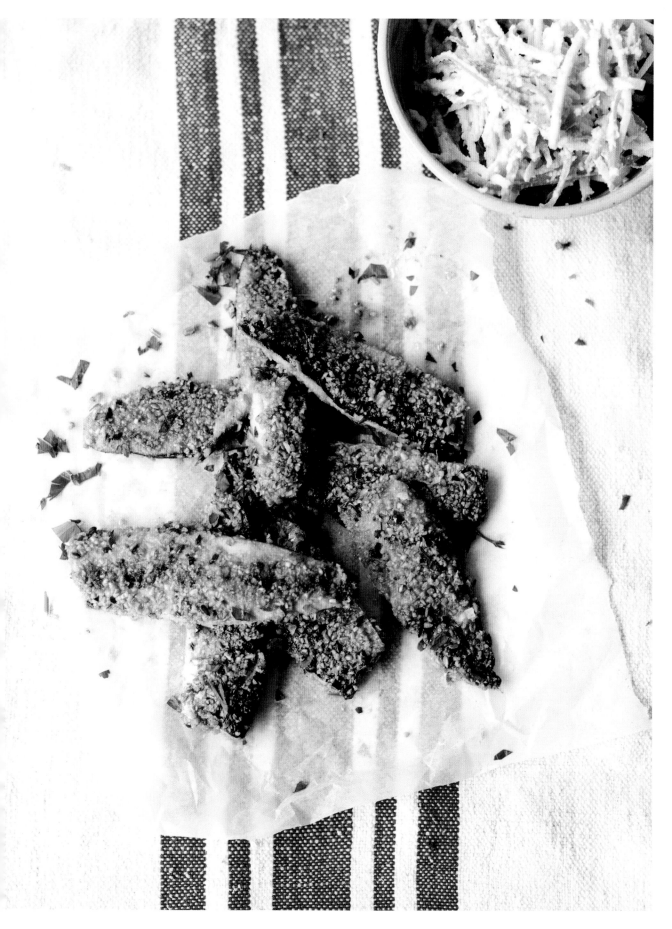

SEAFOOD & FENNEL TAGINE WITH SAFFRON AIOLI

1 portion gives you ▶ FAT 27.1g (of which SATURATES 4.5g) ▶ CARBOHYDRATE 19.9g (of which SUGARS 13.2g)
▶ FIBRE 6.9g ▶ PROTEIN 47.8g ▶ SALT 3.4g

Seafood stews are a classic Swedish winter dish, and as winter seems to last for many months in Scandinavia, it's a dish that I'm quite familiar with! The ingredients are so diverse and fresh that a brief perusal of them should excite the senses in all sorts of ways. A dish made for Instagram!

SERVES 2

PREP TIME: 20 minutes

COOKING TIME: 30 minutes

1 tbsp olive oil
1 large onion, chopped
1 fennel bulb, thinly sliced
1cm (½in) piece of fresh root
  ginger, grated
2 garlic cloves, finely chopped

1 medium-hot red chilli, deseeded
  and diced
1 tsp ground cumin
1 tsp ground coriander
½ tsp harissa paste
450–500ml (16–18fl oz) fresh fish
  stock
2 tsp tomato purée
8 vine-ripened cherry tomatoes,
  cut in half

400g (14oz) mixed raw seafood,
  such as prawns, mussels, squid,
  clams
150g (5½oz) firm thick, skinless
  white fish fillets, cut into large
  bite-sized chunks
1 handful of chopped coriander
  leaves
pink or sea salt and cracked black
  pepper

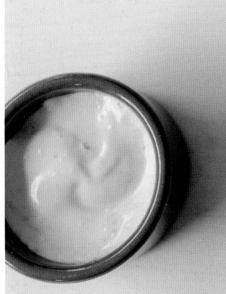

To make the saffron aioli, put the saffron in a ramekin and pour over 1 teaspoon hot water, stir, then set aside for 5 minutes to let it infuse. Put the garlic, egg yolk and mustard into a food processor or blender and blend to a thick paste. With the processor still running, slowly trickle in the oil to make a thick mayonnaise-style sauce. Add the saffron water, season with salt and pepper and spoon it into a serving bowl. Keep the sauce in the fridge until ready to serve.

Now make the tagine. Heat the olive oil in a large, heavy-based saucepan over a medium heat and fry the onion and fennel for 8 minutes until softened. Add the ginger, garlic and chilli and cook, stirring, for another minute before adding the spices, harissa paste, the smaller quantity of stock and the tomato purée.

Stir well and bring to the boil, then turn the heat down to a simmer, part-cover the pan with the lid, and cook for 10 minutes. Add the tomatoes and continue to simmer the sauce, stirring occasionally, for another 5 minutes or until reduced.

SAFFRON AIOLI (SERVES 4–6)

pinch of saffron threads

1 garlic clove, crushed

1 free-range, organic egg yolk

2 tsp Dijon mustard

5 tbsp sunflower oil or light olive oil

pink or sea salt and cracked black
  pepper

bulgur wheat, to serve

Add the seafood and fish and cook, uncovered, for 5 minutes, or until cooked. Add the rest of the stock, if needed, and season with salt and pepper. Scatter over the coriander and serve the tagine with bulgur wheat and topped with a spoonful of aioli.

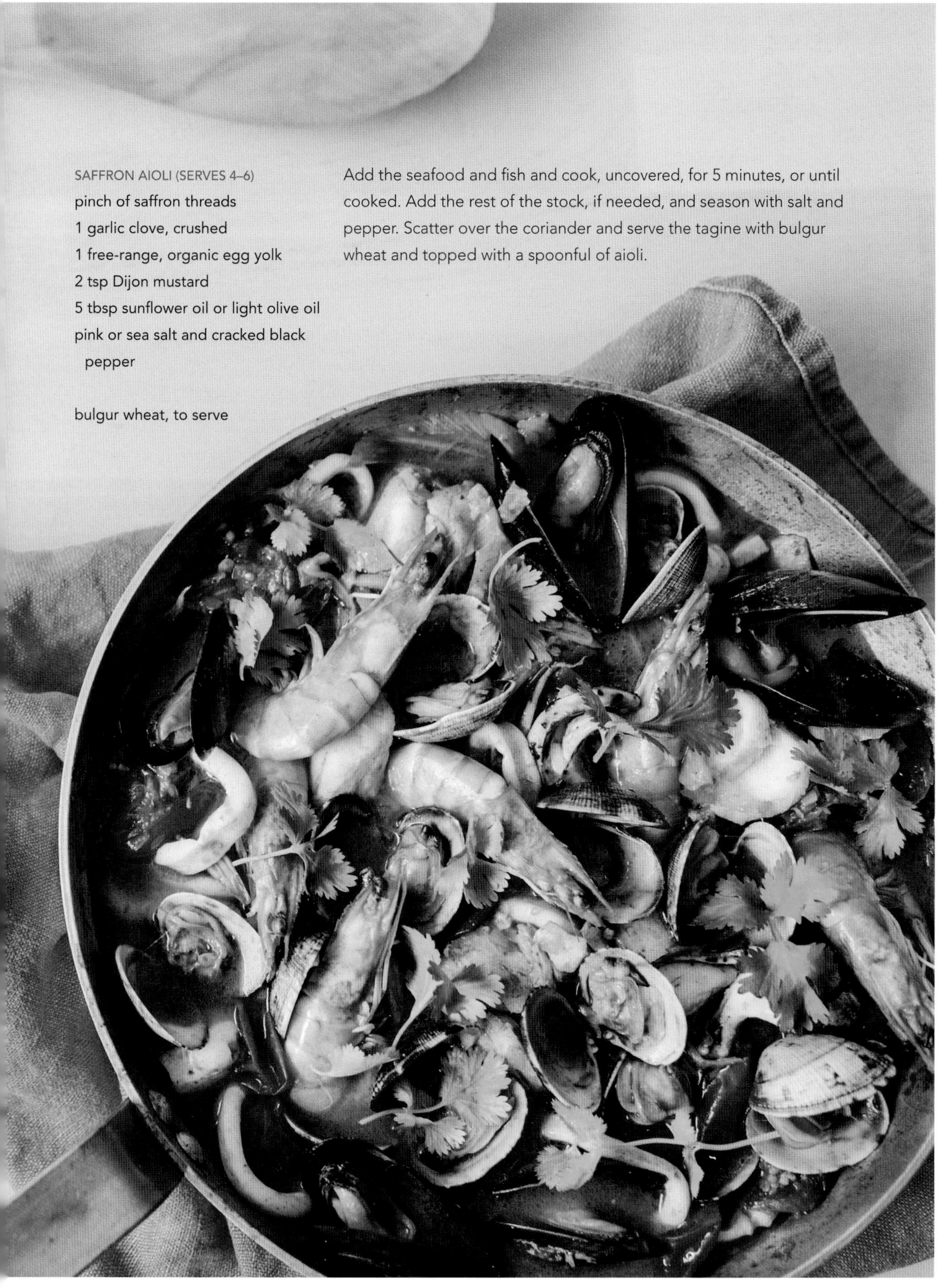

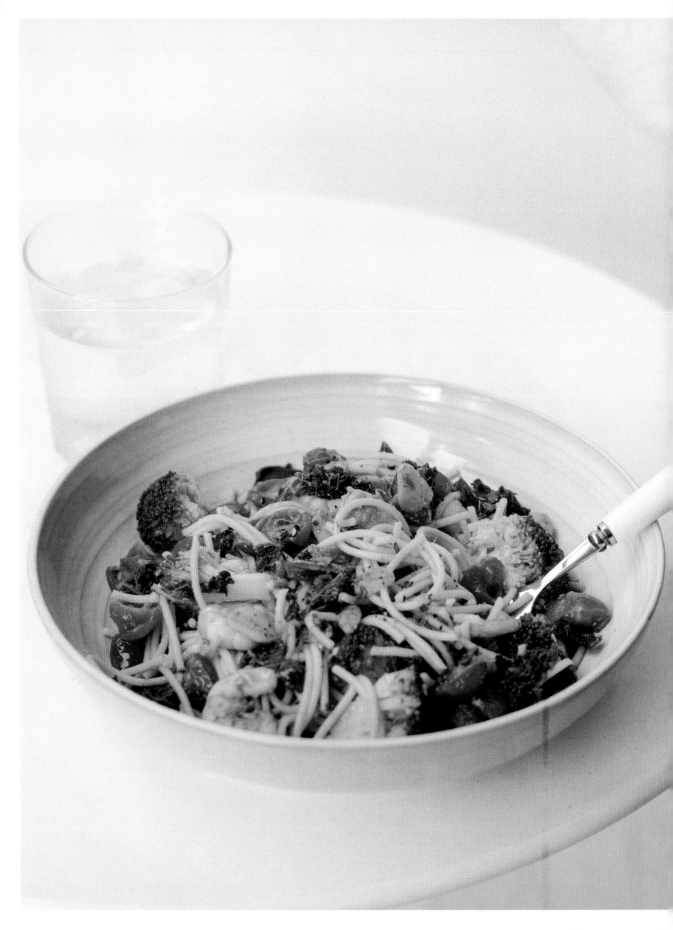

PRAWN, ANCHOVY & GREENS PASTA

1 portion gives you ▶ FAT **19.2g** (of which SATURATES **2.8g**) ▶ CARBOHYDRATE **72.8g** (of which SUGARS **8.5g**) ▶ FIBRE **12.3g** ▶ PROTEIN **50g** ▶ SALT **1.5g**

I'm a huge fan of Italy — it's a disarmingly charming country. My interpretation of a pasta sauce is graced with tomatoes, garlic, prawns and salty anchovies, and garnished with rosemary. Combined, they make for some indulgent comfort food. If you want to opt for some alternatives to wheat pasta, you'll find rice or spelt pastas in your local health-food store. Or, use wholegrain pasta, which is readily available from the supermarkets, and is far better for you than its refined white counterpart.

SERVES **2**

PREP TIME: **15 minutes**

COOKING TIME: **15 minutes**

70g (2½oz) small broccoli florets

70g (2½oz) kale, tough stalks removed and leaves roughly chopped

200g (7oz) brown rice spaghetti or wholegrain spelt spaghetti

1½ tbsp extra virgin olive oil

2 garlic cloves, finely chopped

2 anchovies in oil, drained and finely chopped

1 tbsp finely chopped rosemary

¼ tsp dried chilli flakes

200g (7oz) vine-ripened cherry tomatoes, quartered

225g (8oz) frozen raw king prawns, defrosted (look out for the ones with no added salt)

pink or sea salt and cracked black pepper

Steam the broccoli florets for 2 minutes, add the kale leaves and steam for a further 1 minute, or until both are only just tender. Cool the vegetables under cold running water to stop them cooking any further and to keep their green colour, then set aside.

Cook the pasta in a large saucepan of boiling water following the instructions on the packet until *al dente*.

While the pasta is cooking, put the oil, garlic, anchovies, rosemary and chilli flakes in a large frying pan and heat very gently, stirring frequently, to infuse the flavours in the oil. The anchovies will melt in the heat of the oil.

Add the tomatoes and prawns to the infused oil and cook, stirring, for 2 minutes, then add the broccoli and kale and heat through for another minute, or until the prawns are cooked.

Add 5 tablespoons of the pasta cooking water to the pan to loosen the sauce, then drain the pasta. Add the pasta to the sauce, season with salt and pepper and extra chilli, if you like it hotter, and toss until combined. You're now ready to serve!

SWEDISH CRAYFISH PARTY

1 portion gives you ▸ FAT 12.9g (of which SATURATES 2.8g) ▸ CARBOHYDRATE 32.2g (of which SUGARS 9.7g) ▸ FIBRE 4.2g ▸ PROTEIN 45.2g ▸ SALT 1.1g

In August, Swedes set traps to catch crayfish for the huge national *Kräftskiva* (crayfish party), best enjoyed sitting on a jetty, or in a friend's garden. If you can't find crayfish, use langoustines.

SERVES 2
PREP TIME: **20 minutes**
COOKING TIME: **15 minutes**

1 large bunch of dill
2 tsp fennel seeds or anise seeds
1kg (2lb 4oz) frozen prepared raw
   crayfish or langoustine, defrosted
lemon wedges, to serve
pink or sea salt and cracked black
   pepper

POTATO & RADISH SALAD

375g (13oz) baby new potatoes,
   scrubbed
1 handful of chives, snipped
1 handful of flat-leaf parsley, leaves
   chopped
1 small handful of dill, snipped
5 radishes, chopped
1 tbsp extra virgin olive oil

HERB YOGURT

150ml (5fl oz) plain live yogurt
   or dairy-free alternative
1 small garlic clove, crushed
2 tbsp chopped flat-leaf parsley
   leaves
1 tbsp chopped dill
juice of ½ lemon

Three-quarters fill a large saucepan with salted water and add the dill and fennel or anise seeds, then bring to the boil. Add the crayfish or langoustine, return to the boil and cook for 5 minutes. Strain, then leave the crayfish or langoustine to cool.

To make the potato and radish salad, cook the potatoes in boiling water until tender, then drain and tip them into a serving bowl. Lightly crush the potatoes with the back of a fork, then stir in the rest of the ingredients. Season with salt and pepper.

Mix together all the ingredients for the herb yogurt in a small bowl.

Arrange the crayfish on a serving platter with wedges of lemon around the edge and serve with the potato salad and herb yogurt by the side.

CRAYFISH SONG

The following is just one of the traditional songs we Swedes sing at the annual crayfish festival. It celebrates the beloved crayfish and encourages the revellers to quench their thirst with some warming snaps.

Dom nubbarna, dom nubbarna
är lustiga att ha
Dom nubbarna, dom nubbarna
dom vill vi gärna ha
Ej röra, ej röra, nej skala kräftan först
och sedan, och sedan vi släcka ska vår törst.

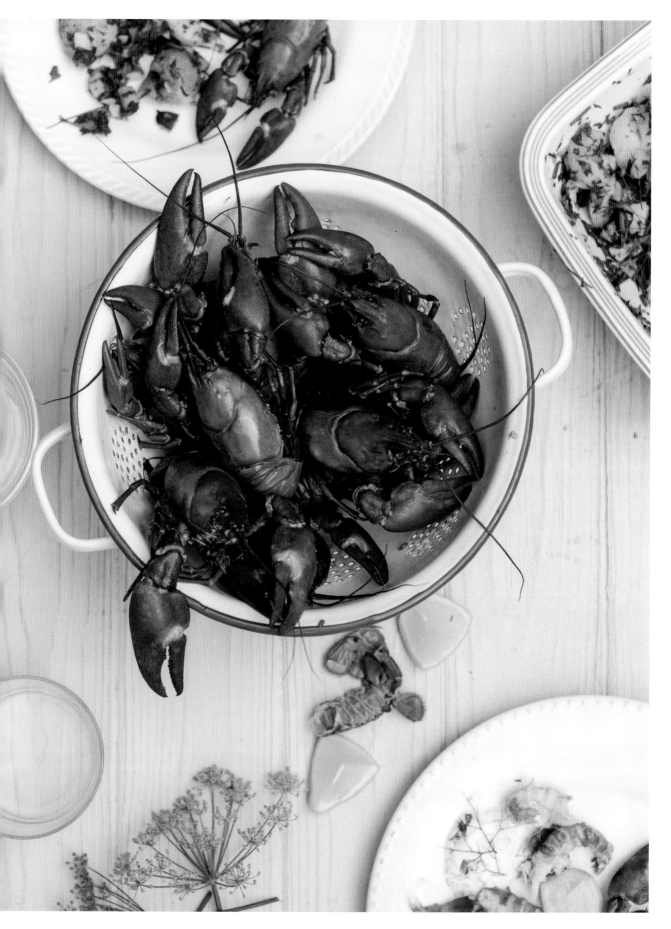

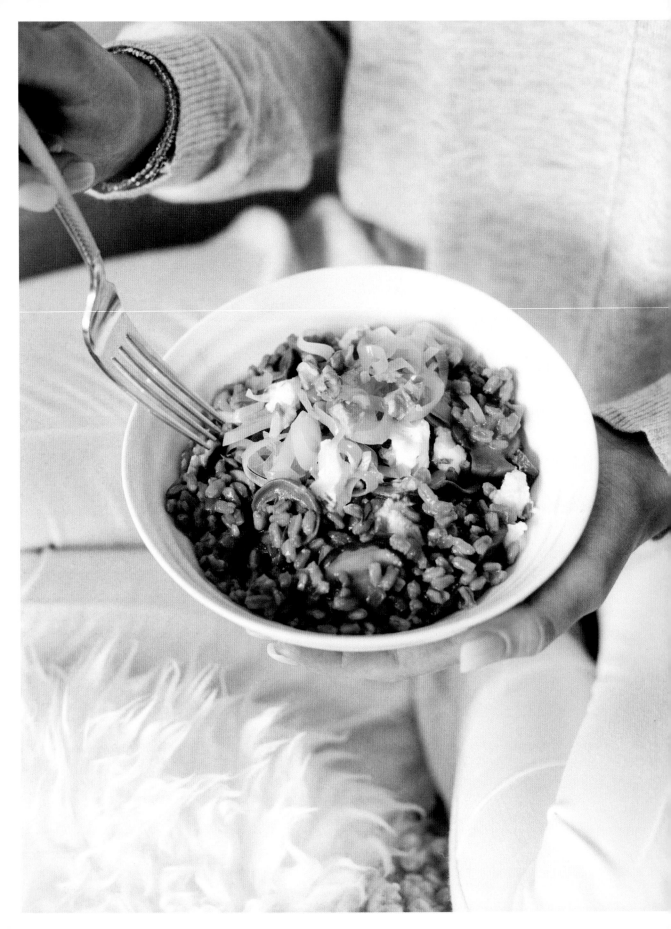

WILD MUSHROOM & SPELT RISOTTO

1 portion gives you ▶ FAT **22.3g** (of which SATURATES **4.9g**) ▶ CARBOHYDRATE **63.4g** (of which SUGARS **9.9g**) ▶ FIBRE **11.5g** ▶ PROTEIN **19.7g** ▶ SALT **1.1g**

Any memories of risotto will likely summon the sensations of richness, fullness of flavour, possibly of excess... With that in mind, I wanted to create something that delivered the same hit of flavour but without the 'risotto oblivion' after-effects. To do that, I found spelt, which is an ancient variety of wheat that contains gluten, but appears to be far better tolerated by those who are otherwise gluten sensitive. It has a slightly nutty flavour, and firm texture a little reminiscent of barley. You add the stock in one go, rather than a ladleful at a time as you would with regular risotto rice. It's an altogether less creamy dish, and somewhat lighter, but no less enchanting!

SERVES **2**

PREP TIME: **10 minutes, plus soaking**

COOKING TIME: **35 minutes**

15g (½oz) dried porcini mushrooms

1 tbsp olive oil

1 onion, chopped

125g (4½oz) chestnut mushrooms, sliced

1 tsp dried thyme

2 garlic cloves, chopped

140g (5oz) pearled spelt, rinsed

275ml (9½fl oz) good-quality, low-salt vegetable stock

25g (1oz) walnut halves

2 leeks, thinly sliced

40g (1½oz) soft goat's cheese, crumbled

pink or sea salt and cracked black pepper

Soak the dried porcini mushrooms in 125ml (4fl oz) just-boiled water for 20 minutes.

When the porcini mushrooms are 15 minutes into their soaking, start preparing the risotto. Heat the olive oil in a large, heavy-based saucepan and fry the onion and chestnut mushrooms for 5 minutes until softened, adding a splash of water to the pan if it gets too dry. Strain the porcini, saving the soaking liquor, tip them into the pan and fry for another 5 minutes until the mushrooms all start to turn golden.

Stir the thyme, garlic and spelt into the pan and cook for 1 minute, stirring, before adding the stock and reserved porcini liquor. Bring up to the boil, then turn the heat down to medium-low and cook, part-covered with the lid and stirring often, for 25 minutes until the spelt grains are tender but have a slight bite. Add more stock, if needed, or take off the lid if the risotto is too wet. Taste and season with salt and pepper, if you need to.

Just before the risotto is ready, toast the walnuts in a frying pan for a few minutes, then leave them to cool and roughly chop. Steam the leeks for 4–5 minutes or until tender.

Spoon the risotto into serving bowls and top with the leeks, walnuts and goat's cheese.

POACHED EGGS ON SMOKY GARLIC CHICKPEAS WITH SMASHED BROAD BEANS

1 portion gives you ▶ FAT 21.6g (of which SATURATES 3.9g) ▶ CARBOHYDRATE 38g (of which SUGARS 16.7g) ▶ FIBRE 13.6g ▶ PROTEIN 25.7g ▶ SALT 1g

The Mediterranean diet is full of splendidly fresh, local and naturally flavoured food, making it healthy by design. This stew will keep in the fridge for up to three days.

SERVES 2

PREP TIME: **20 minutes**

COOKING TIME: **30 minutes**

1 tbsp extra virgin olive oil, plus extra for drizzling

1 large onion, chopped

2 garlic cloves, finely chopped

2 courgettes, quartered lengthways then sliced into chunks

100g (3½oz) drained, canned chickpeas

400g (14oz) can chopped tomatoes

1 tsp hot smoked paprika

1 tsp dried thyme

2 large sprigs of basil

juice of ½ unwaxed lemon, skin reserved

2 large free-range, organic eggs

pink or sea salt and cracked black pepper

SMASHED BROAD BEANS

250g (9oz) shelled broad beans

1 small garlic clove, finely chopped

1 small handful of basil leaves, torn

good squeeze of lemon

drizzle of olive oil

Heat the olive oil in a large, heavy-based saucepan and fry the onion for 5 minutes, stirring regularly. Add the garlic and courgettes and cook for another 3 minutes until the vegetables are tender.

Stir in the chickpeas, tomatoes, spices and herbs and bring almost to the boil. Turn the heat down, add the lemon juice and, for an extra lemony boost, the squeezed-out lemon skin. Simmer, part-covered with the lid, for 20 minutes until reduced and thickened. Season with salt and pepper to taste.

While the stew is cooking, make the smashed broad beans. Steam or boil the broad beans for 3 minutes, or until tender, then refresh briefly under cold running water. Pop them out of their tough outer grey shell to reveal a bright green bean inside, then put them in a mortar with the garlic, basil, lemon juice and a drizzle of olive oil. Roughly crush everything together with a pestle to make a coarse paste, then set aside.

Heat a small pan of water almost to boiling point, turn the heat down and swirl the water. Crack an egg into a cup, then carefully tip it into the gently simmering water and repeat with the second egg. Poach the eggs for a few minutes until the white is set but the yolks are still runny.

Reheat the stew, if you need to, then spoon it into shallow bowls, discarding the lemon skin. Scoop the eggs out of the pan using a slotted spoon and place on top, then finish with a spoonful of the smashed broad beans. Enjoy!

BLINIS WITH ROASTED SPICED CAULIFLOWER

1 portion gives you ▶ FAT 38.3g (of which SATURATES 6.2g) ▶ CARBOHYDRATE 48.1g (of which SUGARS 12.9g) ▶ FIBRE 8.8g ▶ PROTEIN 20.1g ▶ SALT 1.7g

Cauliflower and spices are beautifully suited. Serve the sweet cauli atop a 'dinner-size' blini – or with quinoa, bulgur wheat or brown rice, if no monster blinis are forthcoming.

SERVES **2**

PREP TIME: **20 minutes, plus resting**

COOKING TIME: **30 minutes**

BLINI

50g (1¾oz) buckwheat flour

40g (1½oz) spelt flour

1 tsp baking powder

1 tbsp nutritional yeast flakes

1 free-range, organic egg

100–150ml (3½–5fl oz) unsweetened Homemade Almond Milk (see p.136), or milk of choice

pink or sea salt and cracked black pepper

Fresh Horseradish Cream (see p.93) or Herb Yogurt (see p.100), to serve

SPICED CAULIFLOWER

1 tsp coriander seeds

1 tsp cumin seeds

½ tsp fennel seeds

2 tbsp olive oil, plus extra for frying

2 tsp ground turmeric

large pinch of dried chilli flakes

juice of ½ lemon

150g (5½oz) cauliflower, broken into small florets

1 onion, cut into wedges

1 handful of almonds

First make the blini batter. Mix together both types of flour with the baking powder and nutritional yeast flakes. Whisk the egg in a separate bowl, then gradually beat in the flour mixture, adding enough milk to make a smooth, thick batter. Set aside for 20 minutes to rest, then season with salt and pepper.

Meanwhile, heat the oven to 200°C/400°F/Gas Mark 6.

To make the spiced cauliflower, grind the seeds to a powder in a pestle and mortar, then mix in the olive oil, turmeric, chilli flakes and lemon juice to make a paste. Season with salt and pepper. Put the cauliflower and onion in a bowl, spoon over the spice mixture and turn until the vegetables are evenly coated.

Tip the cauliflower and onion mixture into a roasting tin, spread out in an even layer and roast for 10 minutes. Remove from the oven, scatter the almonds over the top, then return to the oven for another 15–20 minutes until the cauliflower and onion are tender and golden.

While the cauliflower is roasting, heat a large frying pan over a medium heat, then lightly oil the base. Ladle a third of the blini batter into the middle of the pan to make one large blini and cook it for 2–3 minutes on each side until golden. Remove the blini from the pan and cover with foil to keep warm while you make two more (you'll have one spare!).

Serve the blinis topped with the roasted cauliflower mixture and with a spoonful of the horseradish cream on the side.

DESSERTS

As far as I'm concerned, abstinence isn't compatible with happiness. I embrace my cravings for sweetness because satisfying them on a reasonably regular basis keeps me on track with my fitness goals, and keeps me sane. My memories of buying exquisite *kanel bulle* (cinnamon buns) after school have inspired the following desserts. All use delicious ingredients that, while natural and wholesome, totally hit the spot!

(GF) (DF) (V)

KEY LIME PUDDING

1 portion gives you ▶ FAT **20.8g** (of which SATURATES **4.5g**) ▶ CARBOHYDRATE **22g** (of which SUGARS **16.3g**) ▶ FIBRE **6.1g** ▶ PROTEIN **4.7g** ▶ SALT **0.2g**

I make a habit of sampling a slice of Key lime pie when I visit America. This pudding version is lighter, with a refreshing edge; perfect for any summer day, or for accompanying a cup of Earl Grey tea… !

SERVES **2**

PREP TIME: **15 minutes, plus soaking**

150ml (5fl oz) unsweetened
   coconut drinking milk
4 tsp chia seeds
2 pitted dates, finely chopped
½ ripe avocado, stone removed
juice of ½–1 lime, to taste
2 tsp maple syrup (optional)

TO DECORATE
2 heaped tbsp thick unsweetened
   coconut yogurt
finely pared strips of unwaxed
   lime zest
1 handful of blueberries
4 pecan nuts, broken into pieces

Pour the coconut milk into a bowl and stir in the chia seeds and dates. Leave the chia to swell for at least 1 hour, stirring occasionally, or overnight if you have time.

Next, pour the coconut mixture into a blender. Scoop the avocado out of its skin and add to the blender with the smaller quantity of lime juice and the maple syrup, if you like a sweeter pudding. Blend to the consistency of a thick, creamy mousse. Taste and add more lime juice, if needed, or add extra coconut milk if you want a lighter pudding.

Spoon into glasses and top with the coconut yogurt, lime zest, blueberries and pecan nuts to serve.

PASSION FRUIT & COCONUT FRO-YOS

1 portion gives you ▶ FAT 2.3g (of which SATURATES 1.9g) ▶ CARBOHYDRATE 9.6g (of which SUGARS 7.9g) ▶ FIBRE 0.6g ▶ PROTEIN 0.7g ▶ SALT 0.2g

Store-bought ice lollies are replete with added sugars; your fridge can provide the raw materials to make something altogether more delicious and healthy. Start with this creamy yet refreshing popsicle.

SERVES 8

PREP TIME: 10 minutes, plus standing and freezing

2 apples, quartered and cored
2 limes, peeled and halved
8 passion fruits, halved
4 tsp good-quality raw honey
250g (9oz) unsweetened thick coconut yogurt

Juice the apples and limes then pour into a jug. Scoop out the passion fruit using a spoon and stir into the apple and lime juice with the honey.

Pour half of the passion fruit mixture into the ice-lolly moulds, top with the coconut yogurt, then pour in the rest of the fruit mixture until it almost reaches the top of each mould.

Pop in the lolly sticks and freeze for about 5 hours or until frozen. Remove from the freezer about 10 minutes before you want to serve the lollies so they have time to soften slightly. You could dip the top of each one in toasted unsweetened desiccated coconut before serving.

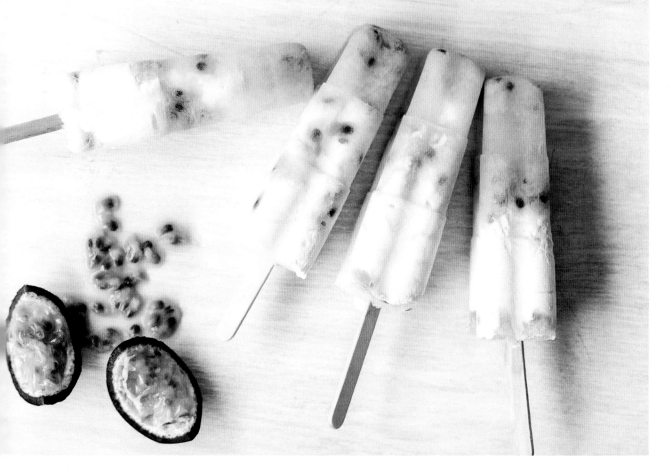

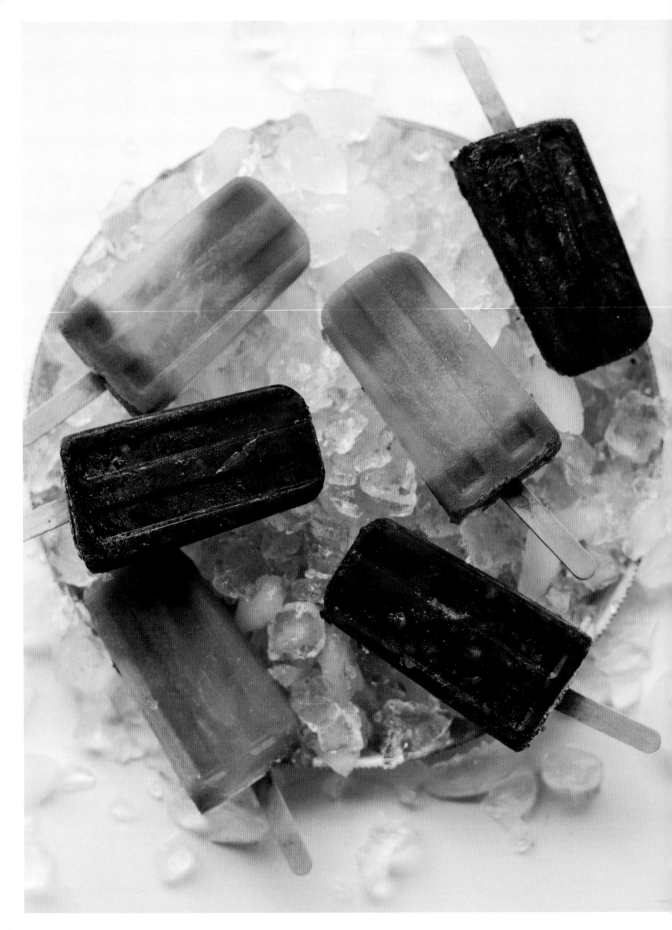

ICE LOLLY BLUEBERRY & BANANA SWIRLS

1 portion gives you ▶ FAT 0.2g (of which SATURATES 0g) ▶ CARBOHYDRATE 9.5g (of which SUGARS 8.3g) ▶ FIBRE 0.6g ▶ PROTEIN 0.4g ▶ SALT 0.003g

Refreshing just to look at, this is an exotic and velvety fruit lolly that will hit the summery spot!

SERVES **4–6**

PREP TIME: **10 minutes, plus standing and freezing**

2 apples, quartered and cored
2 limes, peeled and halved
200g (7oz) blueberries
4 bananas, chopped and mashed

Juice the apples and limes, then pour the juice into a blender with the blueberries and blitz until smooth.

Pour enough of the blueberry mixture into the ice-lolly moulds to fill each one by one-third, top with half of the mashed banana, then continue until the fruit is almost to the top of each mould.

Pop in the lolly sticks and freeze for about 5 hours, or until frozen. Remove from the freezer about 10 minutes before you want to serve the lollies so they have time to soften slightly.

WATERMELON & GINGER SHERBETS

1 portion gives you ▶ FAT 0g (of which SATURATES 0g) ▶ CARBOHYDRATE 3.4g (of which SUGARS 3.3g) ▶ FIBRE 0g ▶ PROTEIN 0.1g ▶ SALT 0.02g

The fiery kick of ginger in these lollies is offset with watermelon's quenching natural sweetness.

SERVES **4–6**

PREP TIME: **10 minutes, plus standing and freezing**

2 apples, quartered and cored
2 limes, peeled and halved
600g (1lb 5oz) rindless, sliced watermelon (prepared weight)
2cm (¾in) fresh root ginger, peeled
2 tsp good-quality raw honey

Juice the apples, limes, watermelon and ginger, then pour into a jug. Stir in the honey and pour the juice into the ice-lolly moulds until it almost reaches the top of each mould.

Pop in the lolly sticks and freeze for about 5 hours or until frozen. Remove from the freezer about 10 minutes before you want to serve the lollies so they have time to soften slightly.

BLACK FOREST CHIA

1 portion gives you ▶ FAT **7.1g** (of which SATURATES **3.1g**) ▶ CARBOHYDRATE **23.4g** (of which SUGARS **20g**) ▶ FIBRE **5.9g** ▶ PROTEIN **5.4g** ▶ SALT **0.2g**

This is a supreme concoction, featuring all the indulgent, sumptuously rich elements of a classic chocolate-and-cherry Black Forest gâteau, and reimagining them in a much healthier format. I'm leaning on chia's superpowers – these super-seeds carry the dish perfectly, and will likely leave you wanting a second helping… Enjoy!

SERVES **2**

PREP TIME: **15 minutes, plus soaking**

100ml (3½fl oz) unsweetened Homemade Almond Milk (see p.136), or milk of choice

4 tsp chia seeds

2 pitted dates, finely chopped

½ tbsp raw cacao powder

1 tsp good-quality vanilla extract

125g (4½oz) fresh dark cherries, pitted

TO DECORATE

2 heaped tbsp Greek live yogurt or dairy-free alternative

¼ tsp ground cinnamon

1 tsp cacao nibs

2 fresh dark cherries

Pour the almond milk into a bowl and stir in the chia seeds and dates. Leave the chia to swell for at least 1 hour, stirring occasionally, or overnight if you have time.

Pour the almond mixture into a blender. Add the cacao powder, vanilla and cherries and blend to a smooth, thick, mousse-like consistency. Add extra almond milk if the mixture is too thick.

Spoon into glasses and top with the yogurt, cinnamon, cacao nibs and cherries.

CHAI CHIA

1 portion gives you ▶ FAT **6g** (of which SATURATES **2.3g**) ▶ CARBOHYDRATE **26.3g** (of which SUGARS **18.6g**)
▶ FIBRE **6g** ▶ PROTEIN **5.1g** ▶ SALT **0.3g**

No, it's not a typo! Chai is traditionally an Indian spiced milky tea flavoured with all sorts of delicious spices, the likes of cardamom, cinnamon, cloves and ginger. You might have encountered it in the form of a chai latte, popularised by many high street café chains. My twist on this classic uses matcha green tea powder (you could also use ground Japanese green tea) instead of the more usual black tea. It's a titan of digestive benefits, and is rich in antioxidant compounds, far more than regular green tea.

SERVES **2**

PREP TIME: **10 minutes, plus soaking/ infusing**

COOKING TIME: **5 minutes**

200ml (7fl oz) unsweetened
  Homemade Almond Milk
  (see p.136), or milk of choice
2 cardamom pods, split
1 cinnamon stick
6 cloves
1cm (½in) piece of fresh root
  ginger, sliced into rounds
4 tsp chia seeds
2 small bananas, sliced
1 tsp good-quality vanilla extract
1–2 tsp matcha tea powder

TO DECORATE
2 heaped tbsp thick unsweetened
  coconut yogurt
Chopped pistachio nuts

Pour half of the milk into a small saucepan and stir in all of the spices. Warm gently for 5 minutes, then turn off the heat, pour the spiced milk into a bowl and leave to infuse for at least 1 hour, or overnight – the longer you leave it the better.

Pour the remaining milk into a bowl and stir in the chia seeds. Leave the chia to swell for at least 1 hour, stirring occasionally, or overnight if you have time.

Strain the spiced milk into a blender, add the chia milk, three-quarters of the bananas, the vanilla and 1 teaspoon matcha, then blend until smooth and creamy. Add extra almond milk if the mixture is too thick, then taste and stir in the extra matcha, if preferred.

Spoon into glasses and top with the coconut yogurt, the remaining sliced banana and the pistachios.

VEGAN MOCHA MOUSSE CAKE

1 portion gives you ▶ FAT **15.8g** (of which SATURATES **5.6g**) ▶ CARBOHYDRATE **22.5g** (of which SUGARS **14.5g**) ▶ FIBRE **4.2g** ▶ PROTEIN **6.6g** ▶ SALT **0.1g**

This rapturous slice of chocolate ecstasy is a 'secret weapon' dessert. Who would ever guess it contains borlotti beans?! It has an oaty nut base topped with an incredibly rich mocha mousse. A thin sliver is all you need – but, it's so worth it!

SERVES: **10–12**

PREP TIME: **30 minutes, plus freezing**

OAT & NUT CRUST

1 tbsp coconut oil, plus extra for greasing

100g (3½oz) hazelnuts

55g (2oz) jumbo porridge oats

55g (2oz) sunflower seeds

4 pitted dates, chopped

1 heaped tbsp peanut butter

1 tbsp date syrup

pinch of pink or sea salt

MOCHA MOUSSE FILLING

100g (3½oz) plain chocolate, about 85% cocoa

400g (14oz) tin borlotti beans, drained and rinsed

4 tbsp espresso coffee

6 pitted dates, chopped

4 tbsp hazelnut milk, or nut milk of choice

2 tsp good-quality vanilla extract

1 tsp ground cinnamon

1 tbsp coconut oil

2 tbsp date syrup

2 bananas, sliced

fresh blackberries, to decorate

Line the base of a 20cm (8in) loose-bottomed tart tin with baking paper and lightly grease the sides with coconut oil.

Start by making the crust. Put the hazelnuts in a large, dry frying pan and toast for 3 minutes, tossing the pan until they start to colour. Tip out of the pan and set aside 40g (1½oz) of the nuts to decorate the cake at the end. Put the rest of the hazelnuts in a food processor.

Put the oats in the pan and toast over a gentle heat for 2–3 minutes, tossing the pan frequently, until starting to turn golden, then tip them into the processor with the nuts. Add the rest of the crust ingredients and pulse a few times until you have a coarse crumb consistency.

Tip the crumb mixture into the prepared tin and press the mixture down with your fingers into a firm, even layer. Put in the freezer while you make the filling.

Melt the chocolate in a heatproof bowl placed over a pan of gently simmering water – do not let the bottom of the bowl touch the water – then leave the melted chocolate to cool slightly.

Put the rest of the filling ingredients in the cleaned food processor, add the melted chocolate and blend for a minute or so until smooth and creamy. Pour the filling on top of the crust, return the tin to the freezer and freeze until the top is firm, about 4 hours.

Take the mousse cake out of the freezer about 30 minutes before serving to allow it to soften slightly. Remove the sides of the tin as soon as you take it out so the filling keeps its shape.

Roughly chop the reserved hazelnuts and scatter over the top with the berries, to decorate. If you don't eat all of the cake straight away, return it to the freezer to firm up again.

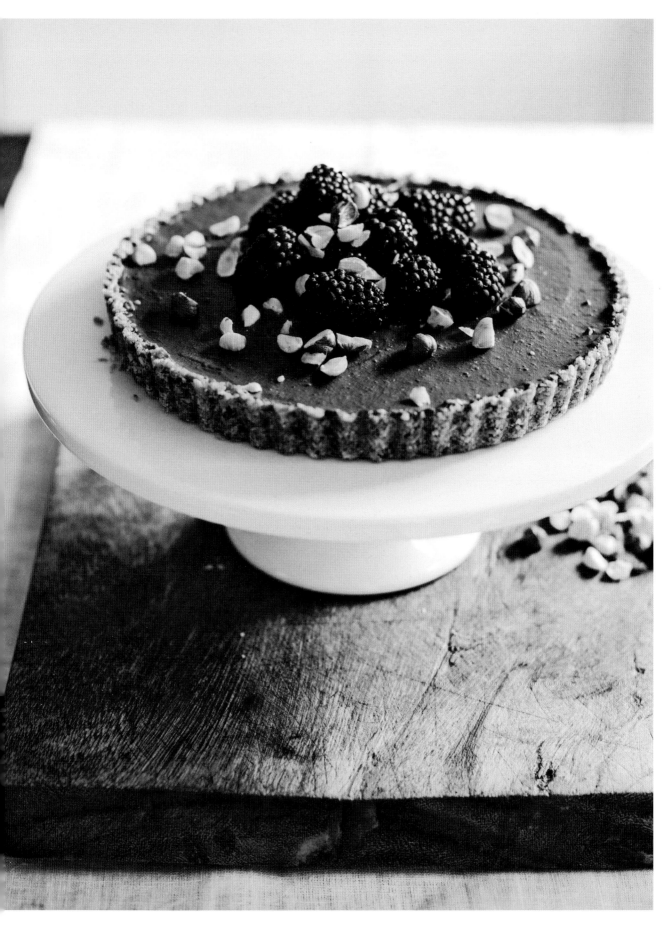

PANCAKE DAY SWEET POTATO RÖSTI WITH FRESH STRAWBERRY JAM

1 portion gives you ▶ FAT **8.8g** (of which SATURATES **3.8g**) ▶ CARBOHYDRATE **23.1g** (of which SUGARS **14g**) ▶ FIBRE **5g** ▶ PROTEIN **13.4g** ▶ SALT **1.1g**

Pancakes are a staple in any Swedish household, regularly eaten with a savoury or sweet topping. Instead of usual potato rösti, I've thrown in magical sweet potato as a healthier, lower-GI alternative. Once again, these pancakes are straightforwards to make, including your own jam (way easier than it might sound!). You can use some of the jam for dessert and save the remainder for another time.

SERVES **2**

PREP TIME: **15 minutes, plus standing**

COOKING TIME: **12 minutes**

100g (3½oz) sweet potato, coarsely grated

100g (3½oz) carrot, coarsely grated

1 free-range, organic egg

1 tsp ground mixed spice

pinch of pink or sea salt

coconut oil, for frying

low-fat cottage cheese, to serve

FRESH STRAWBERRY JAM

175g (6oz) strawberries, hulled

2 tsp chia seeds

squeeze of lemon juice

1 tsp good-quality vanilla extract

To make the fresh strawberry jam, purée half of the fruit using a stick blender, then stir in the chia seeds. Leave for 30 minutes, stirring occasionally, or until the seeds swell and the purée thickens. Roughly mash the rest of the strawberries and stir in the lemon juice and vanilla. Stir the chia mixture into the mashed strawberries and set aside to thicken further and become jam-like in consistency.

To make the rösti pancakes, squeeze the sweet potato and carrot in a clean tea towel to remove any excess moisture that would otherwise stop the rösti crisping up when cooking. Whisk the egg, mixed spice and a pinch of salt in a bowl, then stir in the grated vegetables.

Heat enough coconut oil to lightly coat a large frying pan. Add a small amount of the rösti mixture – there's enough to make six – and gently flatten with a spatula into a thin, even layer, about 7cm (2¾in) in diameter (I prefer my rösti thin and crispy). Add the remaining rösti to the pan and fry them over a medium heat for 2–3 minutes on each side until crisp and golden, then drain on kitchen paper.

Serve the rösti topped with cottage cheese and a good spoonful of the fresh strawberry jam.

APPLE & SPICE CUSTARD POTS

1 portion gives you ▶ FAT **7.5g** (of which SATURATES **4.4g**) ▶ CARBOHYDRATE **10.6g** (of which SUGARS **10.6g**)
▶ FIBRE **1.3g** ▶ PROTEIN **4.7g** ▶ SALT **0.3g**

These adorable little custard pots are topped with chunks of baked spiced apple, offset with just a hint of lemon. My preference is to leave the skin on the apple, as it provides valuable fibre and helps to mix up the texture a little, too.

SERVES **2**

PREP TIME: **10 minutes**

COOKING TIME: **35 minutes**

200ml (7fl oz) whole milk or
   Homemade Almond Milk
   (see p.136)
1½ tsp good-quality vanilla extract
2 tsp good-quality raw honey, plus
   extra for drizzling
⅓ tsp freshly grated nutmeg, plus
   extra for dusting
½ cinnamon stick
1 large free-range, organic egg

SPICED BAKED APPLE

1 apple, skin-on, quartered, cored
   and cut into bite-sized chunks
splash of lemon juice, plus
   ½ tsp finely grated unwaxed zest,
   to decorate
½ tsp mixed spice
1 tsp coconut oil

Heat the oven to 180°C/350°F/Gas Mark 4.

To make the custard, put the milk, vanilla, honey, nutmeg and cinnamon in a small saucepan and heat gently until nearly boiling, stirring now and then. Remove the cinnamon stick.

Beat the egg in a mixing bowl, the slowly pour in the spice-infused milk, stirring with a balloon whisk. Strain the custard through a fine sieve into two large ramekins.

Grate a generous amount of nutmeg over the custards and place the ramekins in a small roasting tin. Pour in enough just-boiled water from a kettle to reach halfway up the sides of the ramekins, then place the tin in the oven for 25 minutes, or until the custards have set but are still slightly wobbly in the middle.

While the custards are baking, make the spiced baked apple. Put the apple in a small roasting tin and add a good squeeze of lemon juice, a splash of warm water and the mixed spice. Stir in the coconut oil until everything is mixed together, then bake for 20 minutes, turning once, or until tender and slightly golden.

Spoon the apples on top of the custards and serve sprinkled with the lemon zest.

PEARS WITH STAR ANISE & ALMONDS

1 portion gives you ▶ FAT **21.5g** (of which SATURATES **3.7g**) ▶ CARBOHYDRATE **24.9g** (of which SUGARS **23.8g**)
▶ FIBRE **6.4g** ▶ PROTEIN **7.7g** ▶ SALT **0.3g**

This reinvention of a traditional recipe is my homage to one of the most divine fruits – the white pear. First, the pear takes a long, relaxing bath in water deliciously flavoured with star anise, cinnamon, ginger and vanilla, then we dress it in a robe of fine flaked almonds. Once baked, the pears develop the most heavenly aroma – and their textural profile has become soft and smooth in the middle, yet crispy, sweet and nutty on the outside. Lovely.

SERVES **2**

PREP TIME: **10 minutes**

COOKING TIME: **30 minutes**

150g (5½oz) caster sugar

1 cinnamon stick, broken in half

1 vanilla pod, split lengthways

2.5cm (1in) piece fresh root ginger, sliced into rounds

3 star anise

2 slightly under-ripe pears, peeled, with stalks

4 tbsp flaked almonds

2 tsp good-quality raw honey, plus a little extra to drizzle, if you like

4 tsp low-fat ricotta or soft cheese

1 tsp finely pared orange zest

Heat the oven to 200°C/400°F/Gas Mark 6.

Put the sugar and spices into a smallish pan with 750ml (1¼ pints) water and heat gently until the sugar has dissolved. Submerge the pears in the poaching liquid and simmer gently for 15–20 minutes until glassy looking and tender to the tip of a knife.

Drain the pears and pat dry on kitchen paper, then stand them on a small baking sheet, levelling the base, if necessary. Drizzle all over with honey, then press the flaked almonds all over the outside of the pears. Bake for 10 minutes until the almonds are golden brown.

Serve with the ricotta scattered with the orange zest and an extra drizzle of honey.

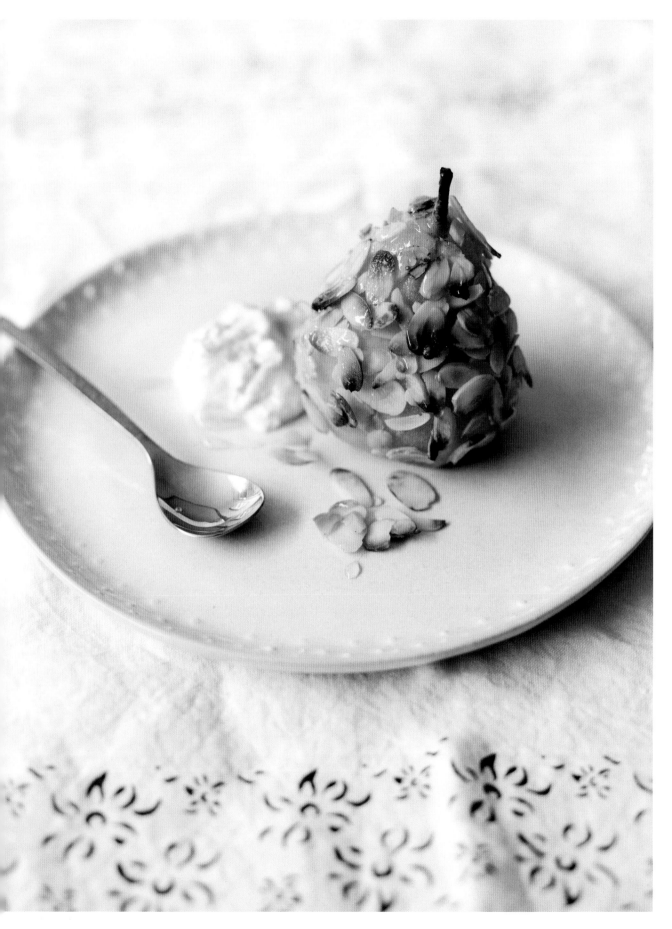

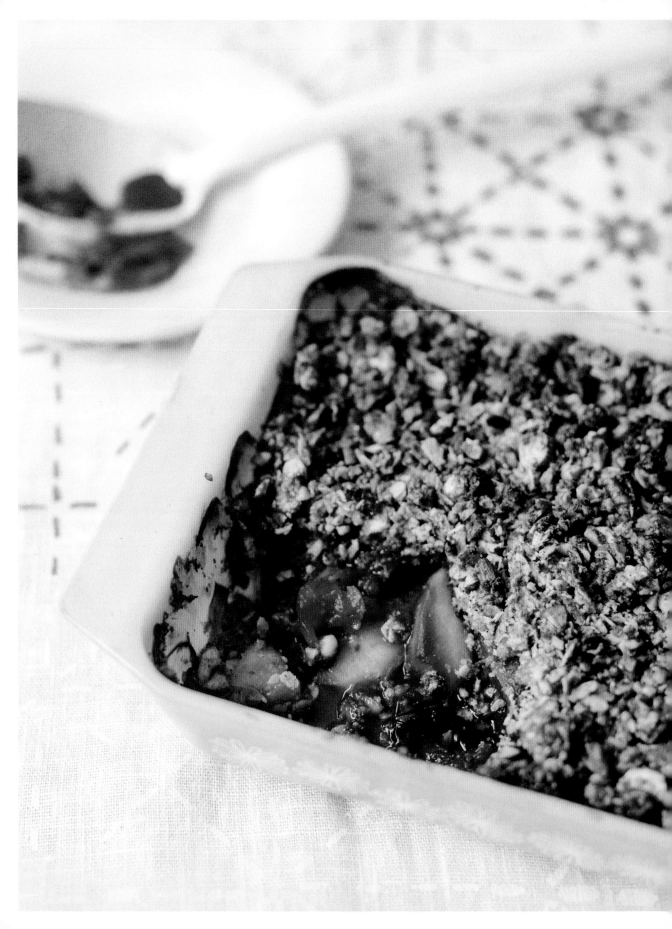

APPLE, RHUBARB & BLUEBERRY CRUMBLE

1 portion gives you ▶ FAT **19.7g** (of which SATURATES **7.9g**) ▶ CARBOHYDRATE **21.6g** (of which SUGARS **11.6g**) ▶ FIBRE **5.3g** ▶ PROTEIN **5.5g** ▶ SALT **0.03g**

What recipe book would be complete without a humble crumble. For some people, a crumble *is* rhubarb crumble; for others it's apple. But I love a good mix, so I've thrown them together and added blueberries. What's more, the crumble topping is gluten-free and vegan friendly. Overall, it's a dessert that will definitely hit the spot.

SERVES **6**

PREP TIME **20 minutes**

COOKING TIME: **45 minutes**

1 large rhubarb stick, cut into 2.5cm (1in) pieces

125g (4½oz) frozen blueberries

1 tsp good-quality vanilla extract

1–2 tbsp good-quality raw honey, to taste

3 eating apples, peeled, cut in half, cored and thinly sliced

CRUMBLE TOPPING

40g (1½oz) hazelnuts, roughly chopped

30g (1oz) almonds, roughly chopped

30g (1oz) pecan nuts, roughly chopped

55g (2oz) jumbo porridge oats

1 tbsp good-quality raw honey

3 tbsp coconut flour

1 tbsp ground cinnamon

3 tbsp coconut oil

Heat the oven to 200°C/400°F/Gas Mark 6.

Start off making the crumble topping as this will allow enough time to chill it before it goes into the oven and that will help make it extra crisp.

Put all the topping ingredients, apart from the coconut oil, in a mixing bowl and stir well until combined. Add the coconut oil and rub it into the crumble mixture, using your fingertips. Pop the crumble topping into the fridge to chill while you prepare the filling.

To make the filling, put the rhubarb and blueberries in a saucepan with a splash of water and cook gently for about 5 minutes until the rhubarb starts to turn mushy. Add the vanilla and enough honey to sweeten. Spoon the apple slices into a shallow 20cm (8in) ovenproof dish and top with the rhubarb mixture.

Take the crumble out of the fridge and scatter it over the fruit filling in an even, chunky layer. Place in the oven for 35–40 minutes, or until the crumble is golden and crisp. Turn the oven down slightly if the crumble darkens too quickly.

SWEET POTATO CHOCOLATE BROWNIES

1 portion gives you ▶ FAT **15.9g** (of which SATURATES **3.3g**) ▶ CARBOHYDRATE **16g** (of which SUGARS **6.1g**) ▶ FIBRE **2.7g** ▶ PROTEIN **5.6g** ▶ SALT **0.2g**

Magic? Witchcraft? A break in the Matrix code? No, it's sweet potato. These gluten-free brownies are provocatively moist, soft and gooey thanks to the addition of the sweet potato, which keeps them molten and delicious. Serve topped with fresh raspberries. Preposterously good.

SERVES **12**

PREP TIME: **15 minutes**

COOKING TIME: **1½ hours**

3 small sweet potatoes, about 600g (1lb 5oz) total weight

100g (3½oz) pecan nuts

coconut oil, for greasing

115g (4oz) almond butter, or nut butter of choice (see p.124)

2 tbsp good-quality raw honey

2 tsp good-quality vanilla extract

40g (1½oz) raw cacao powder

55g (2oz) ground almonds

1 free-range, organic egg, lightly beaten

raspberries, to decorate

Heat the oven to 200°C/400°F/Gas Mark 6. Bake the sweet potatoes for 50 minutes–1 hour until tender. Remove from the oven, cut in half and scoop out the flesh into a mixing bowl – you need about 400g (14oz) in total – and mash until smooth.

At the same time, put the pecans on a baking tray in the bottom of the oven and toast for 10 minutes, turning once, until starting to colour. Leave to cool, then break into large pieces. Line the base of an 18cm (7in) square baking tin and grease the sides with a little coconut oil.

Beat the almond butter, honey, vanilla, cacao powder, ground almonds and egg into the mashed sweet potato until combined. Fold in the pecans, then scrape the mixture into the prepared baking tin.

Bake for 30 minutes, or until cooked through – you want the centre to still be slightly gooey. Leave to cool in the tin, then cut into 12 pieces.

Decorate with fresh raspberries, serve to guests and enjoy the deliciousness with responsible moderation, of course!

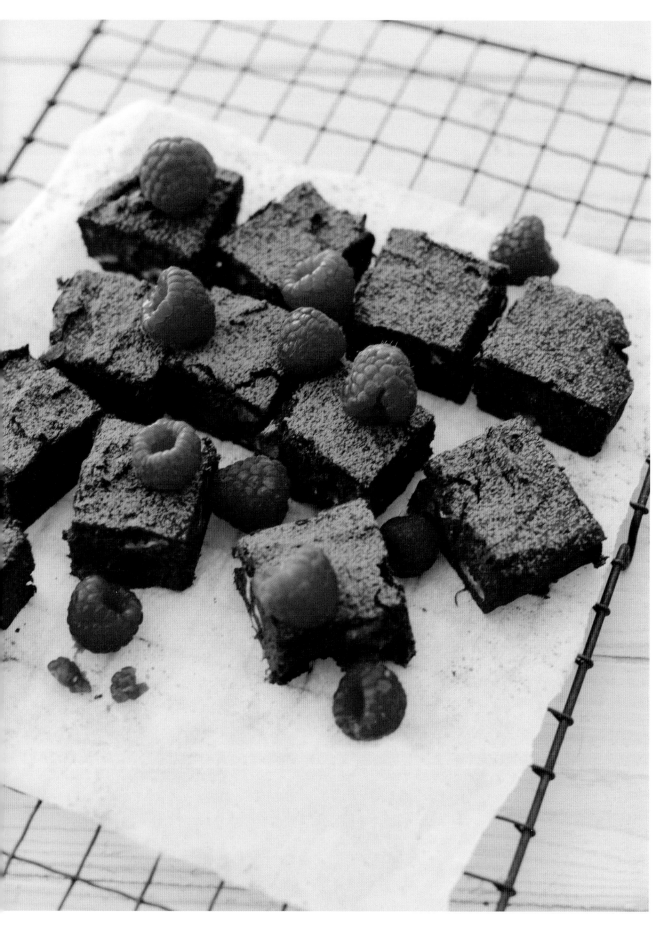

SNACKS

You may think of snacks only as temptations, or naughty treats — but not all snacks are created equal! By eating reasonable portions on a regular basis ('little and often'), and keeping snacks healthy, you'll help to keep your blood sugars and energy levels stable throughout the day. This section includes all my favourite healthy alternatives to chocolate biscuits. They are fabulous snacks without the sugar rush.

GF **DF** **V**

ROASTED SPICED ALMONDS

1 portion gives you ▶ FAT **19.6g** (of which SATURATES **1.8g**) ▶ CARBOHYDRATE **3.1g** (of which SUGARS **1.2g**)
▶ FIBRE **4.4g** ▶ PROTEIN **6.5g** ▶ SALT **0.3g**

The little almond is a giant of nutritional superpowers. To me, almonds are the ideal afternoon snack!

SERVES **2**

PREP TIME: **5 minutes**

COOKING TIME: **15 minutes**

2 tsp olive oil
2 tsp hot smoked paprika or spice
  mix of choice
large pinch of pink or sea salt
85g (3oz) almonds

Heat the oven to 180°C/350°F/Gas Mark 4.

Put the oil, smoked paprika and salt in a mixing bowl. Add the almonds and turn until they are coated in the spiced oil.

Tip the nuts onto a baking tray, spread out evenly, and roast for 10–15 minutes, turning once, until they start to smell toasted and are golden. Leave to cool.

KALE CHIPS WITH ZA'ATAR

1 portion gives you ▶ FAT **7g** (of which SATURATES **2.2g**) ▶ CARBOHYDRATE **2.3g** (of which SUGARS **0.7g**) ▶ FIBRE **3.3g** ▶ PROTEIN **3.4g** ▶ SALT **0.7g**

This foodstuff is basically royalty in terms of 'fitness vogue'; little kale chips take practically no time to make, and if I do say so myself are satisfying, utterly delicious, and offer a bunch of health benefits.

SERVES **2**

PREP TIME: **10 minutes**

COOKING TIME: **15 minutes**

4 large handfuls of curly kale, tough
  stalks discarded and leaves torn
  into bite-sized pieces
coconut oil, for greasing

ZA'ATAR

a few sprigs lemon thyme or
  regular thyme, enough to give
  1 tbsp leaves
1 tbsp sesame seeds
1 tsp sumac
¼ tsp pink or sea salt

Heat the oven to 160°C/325°F/Gas Mark 3. Place the kale on a large baking tray and massage in enough oil with your hands to lightly coat the leaves. Place in the oven and cook for 12–15 minutes, turning the leaves once, until crisp. Keep an eye on the kale as it's prone to burn in the blink of an eye.

While the kale is cooking, make the za'atar. Put the thyme sprigs and sesame seeds on a separate baking tray in the oven for 5 minutes until the leaves are crisp and the seeds start to colour. Remove from the oven, crumble the thyme leaves – discarding the stems – and combine with the sesame seeds, sumac and salt. Leave to cool.

Put the kale in a serving bowl and sprinkle over some of the za'atar. Any leftover spice mix can be stored in a jar for up to 2 weeks – it adds a lemony lift to salads, tagines and soups.

THREE-NUT BUTTER

1 portion gives you ▶ FAT **7.5g** (of which SATURATES **2.2g**) ▶ CARBOHYDRATE **1.7g** (of which SUGARS **0.6g**)
▶ FIBRE **0.8g** ▶ PROTEIN **2.6g** ▶ SALT **0.1g**

It'll be difficult, and take for ever, to do this by hand, so I'd suggest something with a rapid blending motor! Use this yummy nut butter (I've blended three nuts, but you could use a single nut if you prefer) as a dip for sliced fruit, or spread it on a piece of toasted homemade soda bread (see p.129).

MAKES **200g (7oz)**

PREP TIME: **10 minutes**

COOKING TIME: **4 minutes**

100g (3½oz) almonds
50g (1¾oz) peanuts
100g (3½oz) cashew nuts
2 tbsp coconut oil, melted
pink or sea salt

Toast the nuts in a large, dry frying pan for 4 minutes, tossing the pan occasionally, until they start to colour and smell toasted. Rub the nuts in a clean tea towel to remove the brown papery covering, if necessary.

Tip the nuts into a food processor and blitz until finely ground. Add the coconut oil and blend to a smooth, thick paste, occasionally scraping the nuts down the sides of the processor so everything blends evenly. This can take some time and patience – up to 10 minutes – depending on how powerful your processor is.

Season the nut butter with salt to taste and store in an airtight container for up to 2 weeks.

SERVING IDEAS:

▶ For a quick satay sauce or dip, mix together 3 tablespoons Three-nut Butter with 6 tablespoons unsweetened coconut drinking milk, a splash of reduced-salt soy sauce or tamari and a large pinch of dried chilli flakes.

▶ For a delicious chocolatey spread that makes a healthier alternative to popular shop-bought ones, mix together 6 tablespoons Three-nut Butter, 2–3 teaspoons raw cacao powder, 2 teaspoons good-quality raw honey, 2 teaspoons coconut oil and ½ teaspoon ground cinnamon.

▶ Mix together 2 tablespoons of the chocolate-nut spread, above, with enough coconut water to make a dipping consistency. Use as a dip for strawberries or slices of apple, pear or papaya.

▶ Spread a layer of Three-nut Butter or other nut butter over crackers or bread and top with a spoonful of Fresh Strawberry Jam (see p.114).

ON-THE-GO POWER BARS

1 portion gives you ▶ FAT **17.4g** (of which SATURATES **7.1g**) ▶ CARBOHYDRATE **15.5g** (of which SUGARS **5.6g**)
▶ FIBRE **3.1g** ▶ PROTEIN **5.3g** ▶ SALT **0.08g**

When you need a quick snack to deliver a nourishing energy hit, these beauties are perfect, and best of all they fit into your handbag for on-the-go! Make them in bulk and store them in the 'delectable things' cupboard to dispatch when needed!

MAKES **16 squares**

PREP TIME: **15 minutes**

COOKING TIME: **40 minutes**

4 tbsp coconut oil, plus extra for greasing

70g (2½oz) hazelnuts

85g (3oz) cashew nuts

140g (5oz) jumbo porridge oats

40g (1½oz) unsweetened flaked coconut

70g (2½oz) pumpkin seeds, roughly chopped

70g (2½oz) sunflower seeds

½ tbsp ground cinnamon

4 tbsp cacao nibs

100ml (3½fl oz) good-quality raw honey

2 tsp good-quality vanilla extract

pinch of pink or sea salt

Heat the oven to 180°C/350°F/Gas Mark 4. Line the base of a square 23cm (9in) baking tin with baking paper and grease the sides with coconut oil.

Toast the hazelnuts and cashews on a baking tray in the oven for 10 minutes, tossing the nuts halfway, until they smell toasted and start to turn golden. At the same time, toast the oats for 6 minutes. Remove the nuts and oats from the oven, tip them into a food processor and blitz to a coarse powder.

Next, toast the coconut for 4 minutes until crisp and starting to colour. Tip the coconut into a mixing bowl and crush it a little in your hands. Add the nut and oat mixture, the seeds, cinnamon, cacao nibs and a pinch of salt.

Gently heat the coconut oil and honey until melted, then pour it into the nut mixture with the vanilla. Stir until everything is mixed together really well, then tip the mixture into the prepared tin and press down into a firm, even layer with the back of a spoon.

Bake for 22–25 minutes until golden and firm, then leave to cool in the tin before turning out and cutting into 16 small squares.

GF DF V

ENERGY BALLS

1 portion gives you ▶ FAT **4.5g** (of which SATURATES **1.2g**) ▶ CARBOHYDRATE **5.3g** (of which SUGARS **4.5g**) ▶ FIBRE **1.8g** ▶ PROTEIN **1.4g** ▶ SALT **0.01g**

These sumptuous spheres pack a powerfully nutritious punch, and a hit of energy thanks to a dash of espresso coffee. They're great for a pre-workout boost if you need one, and they'll keep you going faster and harder when the going gets tough.

MAKES **20**

PREP TIME: **20 minutes**

COOKING TIME: **6 minutes**

50g (1¾oz) pecan nuts

50g (1¾oz) almonds

150g (5½oz) dried figs, chopped, stalks discarded

3 tbsp espresso coffee (or swap with fresh orange juice)

finely grated zest of 1 orange

2 tbsp cacao nibs

15g (½oz) unsweetened desiccated coconut

15g (½oz) plain chocolate, 85% cocoa, finely grated, or raw cacao powder

Toast the pecans in a large, dry frying pan over a medium-low heat for 3 minutes, turning once, until they start to colour. Tip them into the bowl of a food processor. Toast the almonds in the same way, then add them to the pecans and blitz until very finely chopped. Tip the nuts into a mixing bowl.

Put the figs and coffee into the processor and blend to a paste, then scrape the mixture into the bowl and add the orange zest and cacao nibs. Stir until everything is mixed to a coarse paste.

Cover one plate with the desiccated coconut and a second plate with the grated chocolate or cacao powder. Form the fig paste into 20 balls, each about the size of a large marble, then roll 10 balls in the coconut and 10 balls in the chocolate. Chill in the fridge to firm up until ready to eat – they are best stored in the fridge, too.

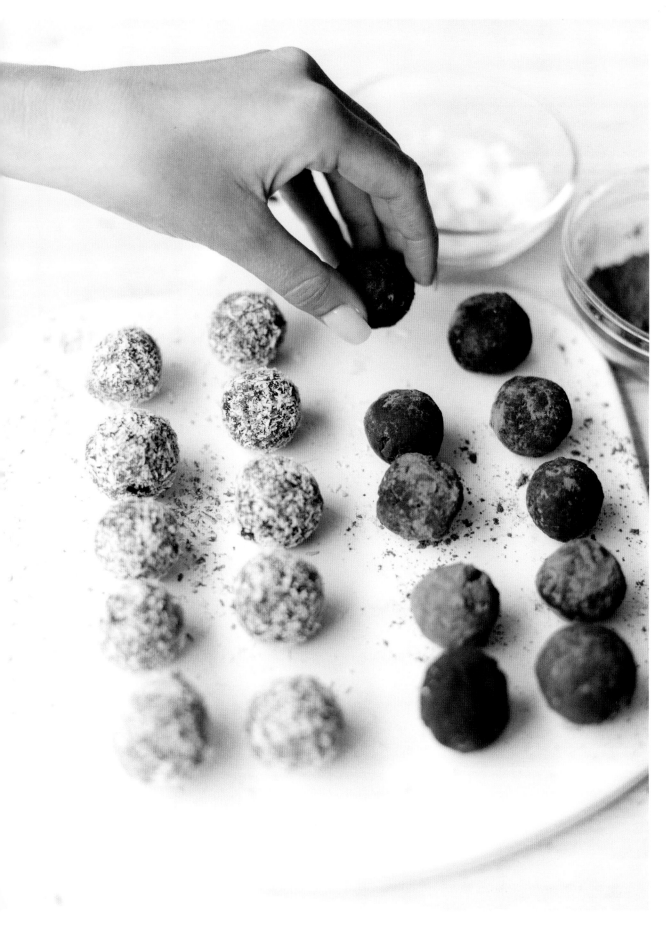

SAVOURY EGG MUFFINS

1 portion gives you ▶ FAT 30.7g (of which SATURATES 6.8g) ▶ CARBOHYDRATE 5.6g (of which SUGARS 2.4g) ▶ FIBRE 5.2g ▶ PROTEIN 31.1g ▶ SALT 2.9g

One observation I've made during my pursuit of a healthy lifestyle is that, often, the concept of 'presentation' just gets totally overlooked. I'd argue that these nutritious little muffins are a perfect example of how mouthwatering presentation can be pretty quick, clocking in at a mere 10 minutes!

SERVES 2

PREP TIME: **10 minutes**

COOKING TIME: **18 minutes**

coconut or olive oil, for greasing

70g (2½oz) frozen petit pois

4 tbsp snipped chives

2 broccoli florets, finely chopped, stalks saved for another dish

4 free-range, organic eggs, lightly beaten

pink or sea salt and cracked black pepper

TO SERVE

slices of smoked salmon or trout

slices of avocado

squeeze of lemon

Heat the oven to 180°C/350°F/Gas Mark 4. Line the base of an 8-hole muffin tin with a round of baking paper and grease the sides with oil.

Cook or defrost the peas until tender. Drain, if necessary, and mash with the back of a fork in a jug. Stir in the chives, broccoli florets and the eggs. Season with salt and pepper and beat until combined.

Pour the pea and egg mixture into the prepared muffin tin and bake for 16–18 minutes until the egg muffins have risen and started to turn golden. Wait for a few minutes, run a knife around the edge of each muffin and lift them out of the tin.

Top four of the muffins with a slice of salmon or trout, sliced avocado and a squeeze of lemon. Then top with a second egg muffin to make four egg muffin 'sandwiches'.

SPELT & QUINOA SODA BREAD

1 portion gives you ▶ FAT **4.8g** (of which SATURATES **0.7g**) ▶ CARBOHYDRATE **32g** (of which SUGARS **3g**) ▶ FIBRE **3.2g** ▶ PROTEIN **9.2g** ▶ SALT **0.9g**

Bread-making is so much easier than you may think and the uplifting aroma of it, freshly baked, sweeping majestically out of the oven is truly heroic. To celebrate your accomplishment, top this special soda bread with some of my homemade fresh strawberry jam or nut butter for a yummy snack.

MAKES **1 x 450g (1lb) loaf**

PREP TIME: **10 minutes**

COOKING TIME: **45 minutes**

375g (13oz) wholegrain spelt flour, plus extra for dusting

70g (2½oz) quinoa flour

1 tsp pink or sea salt

1 tsp bicarbonate of soda

3 tbsp sunflower seeds

2 tbsp ground flaxseeds

400ml (14fl oz) buttermilk (or plain yogurt mixed with 1 tbsp lemon juice)

Heat the oven to 200°C/400°F/Gas Mark 6 and dust a baking sheet with a little flour.

Sift the spelt flour, quinoa flour, salt and bicarbonate of soda into a mixing bowl. Stir in the sunflower seeds and flaxseeds and make a well in the middle.

Pour the buttermilk into the bowl and gently mix with outstretched fingers to make a soft, slightly sticky dough.

Tip the dough out onto a lightly floured work surface and gently knead it into a smooth ball – try not to over-work it or the bread will be heavy. Place the dough on the floured baking tray and press it down with the palm of your hand until it's about 5cm (2in) high.

Cut a deep cross into the top of the dough and sift a little extra flour over the top. Bake for 40–45 minutes until risen and golden. Tap the base of the bread and if it sounds hollow it's ready. Leave the bread to cool on a wire rack.

JUICES

In this section, you'll find my 'multi-vitamin power-shots'. These little bad boys are packed with vitamins and minerals fresh from the natural source. The reason they're shots and not large glasses of juice is because of the high sugar content. When possible, opt for a cold-press juicer, or squeeze by hand. Many high-speed 'centrifugal' juicers generate such heat as they whiz, they warm up the complex fruit sugars, turning them into less healthy simpler sugars. Cold presses, or masticating juicers, leave behind a cake of fibrous pulp, and pure, unheated, nutritionally intact juice. Yum!

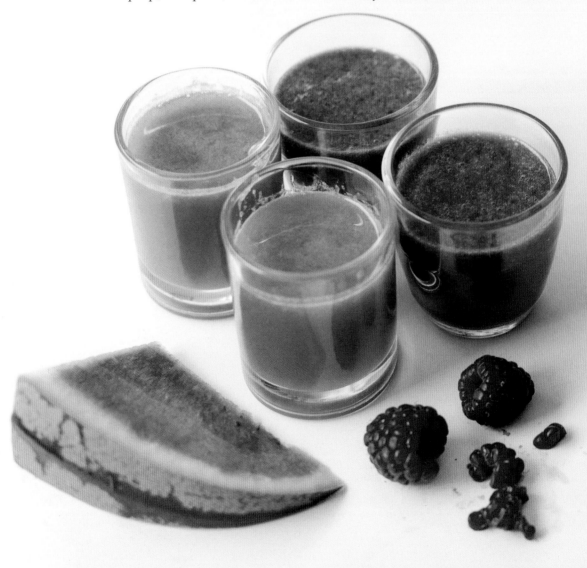

SUPER-VIT

1 portion gives you ▶ FAT 0.1g (of which SATURATES 0g) ▶ CARBOHYDRATE 7.7g (of which SUGARS 5.3g) ▶ FIBRE 0.6g ▶ PROTEIN 1g ▶ SALT 0.06g

A superb multi-vitamin hit, the elegant and refreshing combo of watermelon, ginger and cucumber is up there with my favourite shots to kick off a hot, summer day, or – for that matter – to give me some vigour on a cold winter morning!

SERVES **2**

PREP TIME: **5 minutes**

250g (9oz) rindless, sliced
  watermelon (prepared weight)
½ lime, peeled
1cm (½in) piece of fresh root
  ginger, peeled
8cm (3¼in) piece of cucumber,
  quartered lengthways

Juice the watermelon, lime, ginger and cucumber, then pour the juice into two small glasses and serve straight away.

ROCKET FUEL

1 portion gives you ▶ FAT 0.6g (of which SATURATES 0g) ▶ CARBOHYDRATE 9.8g (of which SUGARS 5.1g) ▶ FIBRE 1.2g ▶ PROTEIN 1.9g ▶ SALT 0.03g

While it won't send you into orbit, the combination of these sweet, sour and tangy ingredients creates a flavour explosion, which will certainly help launch the day with a mineral boost!

SERVES **2**

PREP TIME: **5 minutes**

2 handfuls of raspberries
2 handfuls of kale
1 lemon, peeled
½ orange, peeled
1 handful of parsley sprigs

Juice the raspberries, kale, lemon, orange and parsley, then pour the juice into two small glasses and serve straight away.

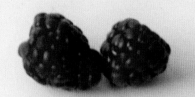

ENERGISER

1 portion gives you ▶ FAT 0.1g (of which SATURATES 0g) ▶ CARBOHYDRATE 9.4g (of which SUGARS 7.1g) ▶ FIBRE 0.4g ▶ PROTEIN 0.4g ▶ SALT 0.02g

This little energy-booster is great when you need some zing to carry you into the day.

SERVES **2**

PREP TIME: **5 minutes**

100g (3½oz) sweet potato, peeled
   and cut into long wedges
1 apple, quartered and cored
1 lime, peeled
1cm (½in) piece of fresh root
   ginger, peeled

Juice the sweet potato, apple, lime and ginger, then pour the juice into two small glasses and serve straight away.

PURPLE VITALITY

1 portion gives you ▶ FAT 0.2g (of which SATURATES 0g) ▶ CARBOHYDRATE 5.1g (of which SUGARS 3.3g) ▶ FIBRE 0.7g ▶ PROTEIN 0.9g ▶ SALT 0.04g

The beetroot delivers a gorgeous purple hue, as well as providing a succulent and sweet flavour in this energy shot.

SERVES **2**

PREP TIME: **5 minutes**

1 small raw beetroot, quartered
100g (3½oz) blueberries
1cm (½in) piece of fresh root
   ginger, peeled
1 large handful of kale
½ lemon, peeled

Juice the beetroot, blueberries, ginger, kale and lemon, then pour the juice into two small glasses and serve straight away.

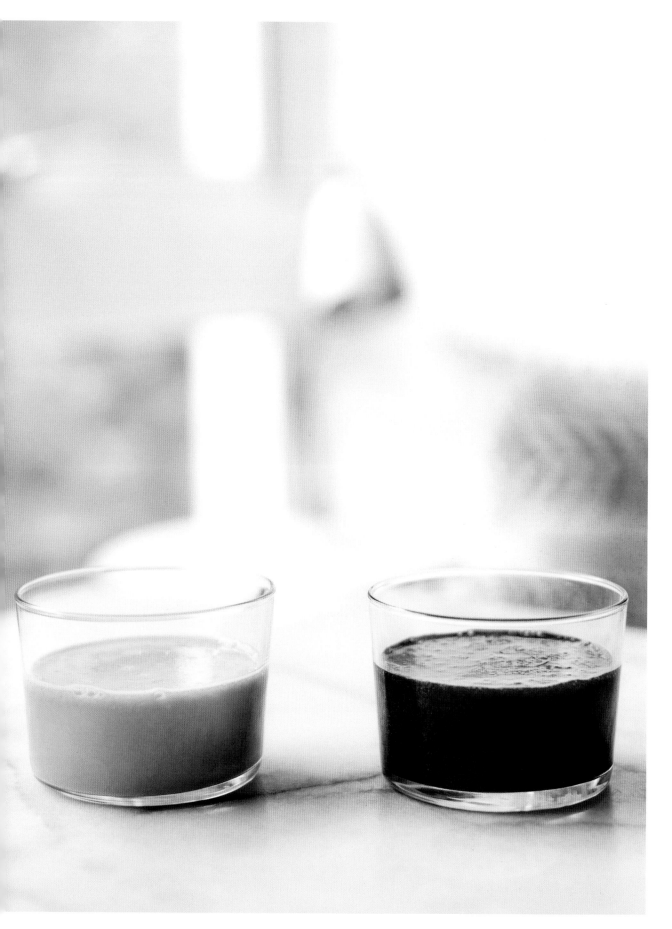

VITAMIN-C BOMB

1 portion gives you ▶ FAT 0.1g (of which SATURATES 0.1g) ▶ CARBOHYDRATE 3.6g (of which SUGARS 3.3g)
▶ FIBRE 0.1g ▶ PROTEIN 0.4g ▶ SALT 0.02g

Refreshing and sweet, loaded with mineral goodness, the clue is in the name: this shot is a great source of vitamin C to help ward off coughs and colds.

SERVES **2**

PREP TIME: **5 minutes**

1 large orange, peeled and
   quartered
1 small raw beetroot, quartered
1cm (½in) piece of fresh root
   ginger, peeled
½ lemon, peeled
1cm (½in) turmeric root or
   ½ tsp ground turmeric

Juice the orange, beetroot, ginger, lemon and turmeric (or stir in the turmeric powder at the end). Pour the juice into two small glasses and serve straight away.

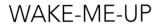

WAKE-ME-UP

1 portion gives you ▶ FAT 0.2g (of which SATURATES 0g) ▶ CARBOHYDRATE 7.7g (of which SUGARS 6.5g)
▶ FIBRE 0g ▶ PROTEIN 0.7g ▶ SALT 0.06g

This is a refreshing, tangy yet sweet juice – fabulous when you need something fresh to start the day.

SERVES **2**

PREP TIME: **5 minutes**

1 apple, quartered and cored
2 handfuls of spinach
1cm (½in) piece of fresh root
   ginger, peeled
½ lime, peeled

Juice the apple, spinach, ginger and lime, then pour the juice into two small glasses and serve straight away.

GF **DF** **V**

IMMUNE BOOSTER

1 portion gives you ▶ FAT 0.2g (of which SATURATES 0g) ▶ CARBOHYDRATE 8.7g (of which SUGARS 8.4g) ▶ FIBRE 0g ▶ PROTEIN 0.4g ▶ SALT 0.05g

Chock-a-block full of vitamins, this juice shot helps to keep your immune system Scandi fit!

SERVES 2

PREP TIME: 5 minutes

2 carrots, halved lengthways
1cm (½in) piece of fresh root
  ginger, peeled
1 apple, quartered and cored
½ lime, peeled
1cm (½in) turmeric root or ½ tsp
  ground turmeric

Juice the carrots, ginger, apple, lime and turmeric (or stir in the powder at the end), then pour the juice into two small glasses and serve straight away.

HOMEMADE MILKS

Entire supermarket shelves are stocked with cow's milk alternatives. Almond and coconut milks are among my favourites. I like the organic process of creating my own, tasting the pulpy imperfections and knowing precisely what's gone into them.

GF **DF** **V**

ALMOND MILK

1 portion gives you ▶ FAT 12.3g (of which SATURATES 0.9g) ▶ CARBOHYDRATE 2.4g (of which SUGARS 1g) ▶ FIBRE 3g ▶ PROTEIN 5.3g ▶ SALT 0.5g

A superb source of monounsaturated fats, almonds are also naturally high in protein, fibre and myriad micronutrients, and yet low in sodium and cholesterol. Making your own almond milk is super-easy!

MAKES **about 400ml (14fl oz)**

PREP TIME: **15 minutes, plus soaking**

100g (3½oz) almonds

400ml (14fl oz) filtered water, plus extra for soaking

pinch of pink or sea salt

Soak the almonds in plenty of filtered water overnight in the fridge.

The next day, drain and rinse the almonds in fresh water. Tip them into a blender with the measured water and salt. Blend for 2–3 minutes on high until the nuts become a fine meal and the water is milky white.

Strain the almonds through a nut-milk bag or muslin-lined sieve over a bowl, squeezing the bag to extract the maximum liquid. Save the leftover meal to use in energy balls, granola bars or muesli mix.

Pour the milk into a lidded jug or bottle and chill for up to 3 days – be sure to stir or shake the milk each time you use as it tends to separate.

RICH ALMOND MILK For a rich, creamy alternative to single dairy cream, reduce the quantity of filtered water to 200ml (7fl oz).

SPICED ALMOND MILK For a comforting drink, warm a cup of almond milk with ½ tsp ground cinnamon, ¼ tsp turmeric, 1 split cardamom pod and ½ tsp good-quality vanilla extract, then discard the cardamom.

COCONUT ALMOND MILK Reduce the water quantity to 300ml (10fl oz) and add 100ml (3½fl oz) coconut water or coconut drinking milk.

COCONUT MILK

1 portion gives you ▶ FAT **21.7g** (of which SATURATES **18.7g**) ▶ CARBOHYDRATE **2.1g** (of which SUGARS **2.1g**)
▶ FIBRE **4.8g** ▶ PROTEIN **2g** ▶ SALT **0.03g**

You can use a fresh coconut to make this creamy milk, but desiccated coconut is perfect and probably more convenient.

MAKES **about 400ml (14fl oz)**
PREP TIME: **15 minutes, plus soaking**

140g (5oz) unsweetened desiccated
  coconut
400ml (14fl oz) filtered water

Put the coconut in a bowl and cover with plenty of filtered water, stir well to make sure all the coconut is submerged, then leave to soak overnight in the fridge.

The next day, strain the coconut and pour away the soaking water. Tip the coconut into a blender with the measured water and blend on high for 2 minutes, or until the coconut is finely chopped and the liquid is creamy white.

Strain the coconut through a nut-milk bag or a muslin-lined sieve over a bowl, squeezing the bag to extract as much liquid as possible.

Pour the milk into a lidded jug or container and store in the fridge for up to 3 days. The coconut meal left in the bag can be sprinkled over breakfast cereal or muesli or added to cookies and cakes.

You'll find the coconut cream rises to the surface – either scrape this off to use separately or stir it in.

HOMEMADE COCONUT CREAM The amount of water you blend with the coconut depends on how thick or thin you like your milk. For an alternative to shop-bought tinned coconut milk to use in curries and sauces, reduce the quantity of filtered water to 200ml (7fl oz).

FRESH COCONUT MILK If you want to use fresh coconut instead of desiccated, crack open the coconut and pour the water into a jug. Chop the coconut into small pieces and cut off the outer brown skin. Make the coconut water up to 400ml (14fl oz) with filtered water and add to a blender with the coconut. Blend on high for 3 minutes until very finely chopped, then leave to soak overnight. The next day, strain through a nut-milk bag or muslin-lined sieve over a bowl, squeezing to extract as much liquid as possible, then pour the milk into a jug.

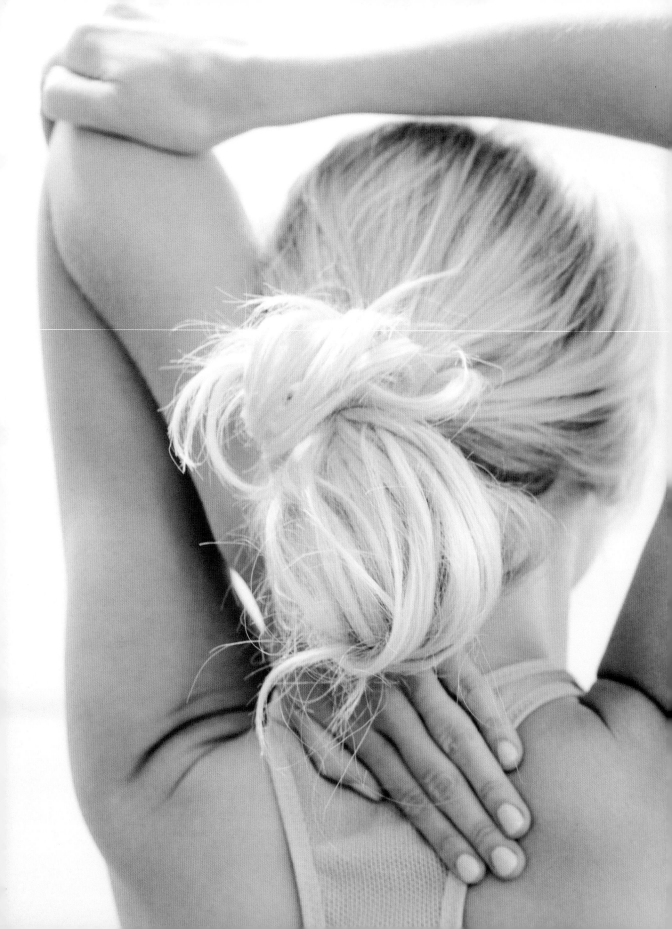

CHAPTER 3

Training
THE Frame

'Gone was the rusty old
hatchback – I had started
to build an altogether
sportier chassis!'

HOW YOUR MUSCLES WORK

In Sweden, I used to run for hours through the ash-tree forests and around the ice-water lakes. Although I loved running, it wasn't until I started to weight train that my running improved – my core and legs felt stronger and my posture improved. I realised then that the whole body works together. Gone was the rusty old hatchback – I had started to build an altogether sportier chassis!

There are some 600 muscles in the body. The way they connect together is mind-bogglingly complex, but knowing the basics of what action a muscle has on a joint can help you to structure your workout.

WHAT DO MUSCLES ACTUALLY DO?

Broadly speaking, there are two types of muscle – the type you're in control of (voluntary) and the type that works all on its own (involuntary). Skeletal muscles (attached to your bones via tendons) are voluntary – by and large, you control them; the visceral muscles (lining the internal organs and blood vessels) and the cardiac muscles (surrounding the heart) are involuntary – they just get on with the job. Aside from holding us upright, stabilising joints and generating heat, muscles do three things:

1 THEY PULL A muscle is like an elastic band that stretches from one bone to another. When a muscle contracts, it creates a pulling motion at the points of attachment, forcing those bones to move. And this is all controlled by your brain. Incredible!

2 THEY WORK TOGETHER There's a beautiful symmetry to the way pairs of muscles (biceps and triceps, quadriceps and hamstrings, and so on) join forces as antagonistic pairs: one muscle contracts as the opposing muscle relaxes. Awesome natural teamwork!

3 THEY TWITCH Muscles react to an electrical current zipping through them at different speeds making some muscles 'slow twitch' and others 'fast twitch'. Long-distance runners have super-developed slow-twitch fibres that are slow to tire – perfect for endurance! Sprinters have bundles of fast-twitch fibres, which contract rapidly for bursts of speed, but which tire at speed, too.

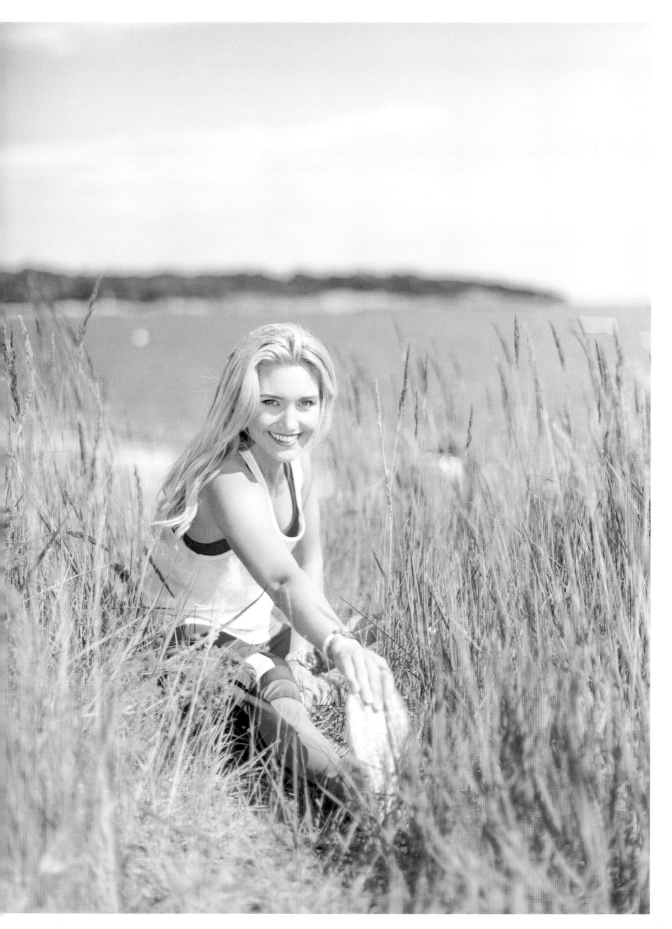

THE MUSCLE ALL-STARS

The following muscles (all of them labelled by corresponding number on the front and back diagrams, opposite) are the all-stars of your body. These are the fibre-packed champs that carry the greatest load when you move, lift, and power-out. We're working through them more-or-less top to toe.

FRONT OF THE BODY

1   DELTOIDS (a) *Medial (middle)*
    (b) *Anterior (front)* Shoulder power!
    You'd engage these when pouring water
    from a jug, or when impersonating Rose,
    arms flung wide, at the front of the *Titanic*...

2   PECTORALS (a) *Major* (b) *Minor* Chest pump!
    You'd engage these when powering a
    forehand down the line during a game of
    tennis, or when pressing yourself up from
    lying face-down on the sun lounger!

3   BICEPS Arms front! You'd engage these when
    lifting your suitcase off the baggage reclaim,
    or your shopping bag from the checkout.

4   ABDOMINALS (a) *Rectus* (b) *Obliques*
    Iron core! You'd engage these when sitting
    up in bed, and then again when lying back
    down to fall back asleep!

5   QUADRICEPS Feel it in those thighs! You'd
    engage these when squatting to sit down,
    or perhaps if you fancy performing the Haka
    like the All Blacks!

BACK OF THE BODY

6   TRAPEZIUS Right at the top! When you
    haven't got a clue and you simply have to
    shrug your shoulders – that's when you're
    using the trapezius!

7   RHOMBOIDS You'd engage these when
    squeezing your shoulders together, as if you
    were trying to hold a stick between them
    (like you do!).

8   TRICEPS Arms back! You'd engage these if
    you were to throw a javelin or, more likely,
    do a press up.

9   LATISSIMUS DORSI Power in your back. You'd
    engage these for gruelling butterfly stroke in
    the swimming pool.

10 GLUTEUS MAXIMUS Butt power! You'd
    engage these when pulling your leg back
    to kick a football.

11 HAMSTRINGS Backs of your legs. You'd
    engage these when transitioning from sitting
    to standing.

12 CALVES Long and lean in the legs! You'd
    engage these when standing on tippy-toes
    to catch a glimpse of Queen Bey at a sell-
    out concert!

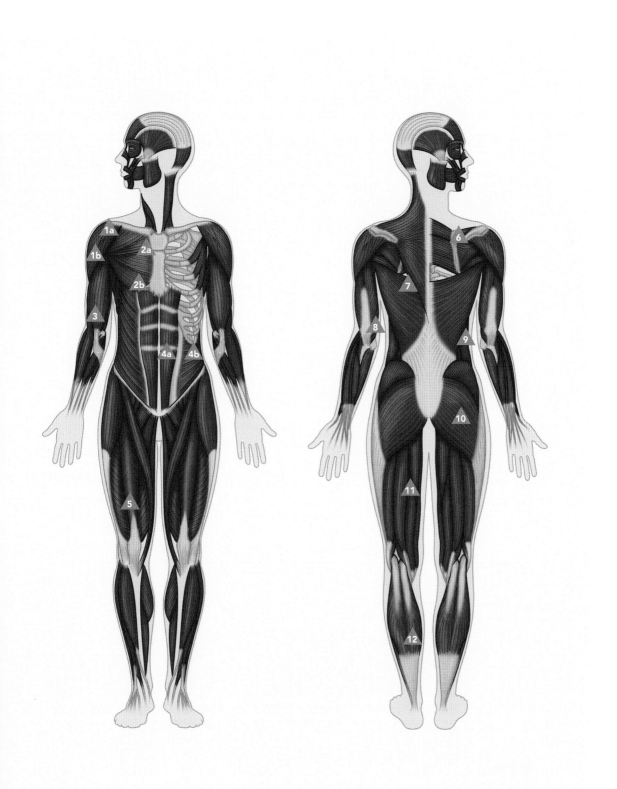

HOW YOU USE YOUR ENERGY: AEROBIC AND ANAEROBIC

Even for those who work out regularly, the difference between aerobic and anaerobic exercise is something most of us remember probably only dimly from school. But an awareness of how our bodies use the fuel we put into them can help us train more efficiently.

THE ANAEROBIC ZONE

You're exercising hard, panting for air and your body can't source enough oxygen to support your muscles. Instead, you burn your sugar (carbohydrate) stores as an immediate source of extra fuel. You're in the ultimate fat-burning zone, accessed via a HIIT session (see p.156) or the likes of 100m sprints (where around 90 per cent of your energy comes from sugar stores), gymnastics, competition fencing, squash, sprint swimming, flipping tyres, battle ropes… generally, any high-intensity activity that requires serious exertion over a short space of time. As with a HIIT workout, mini-recovery sessions will help you return to aerobic operation before toasting calories again on your next burst of activity!

THE AEROBIC ZONE

You're exercising gently, comfortably taking on enough oxygen to supply the muscles; this is 'oxygen surplus' and it feels good. You're consuming blood glucose, glycogen and fat to fuel yourself, but it's more balanced and sustainable energy consumption. The pulse rate is elevated but not rampant, and you can sustain this level of exertion for longer – lucky, because you access this zone via long-distance running, swimming slowly for many lengths, rowing at a moderate pace or going for a lively hike. If your fitness level is low, you can work in your aerobic zone for a while before puffing out and hitting your anaerobic threshold.

Both 'zones' have their place in a well-rounded fitness programme and exactly how you balance them depends on your level of fitness and your fitness goals. In my three-week plan (in Chapter 4), each week provides one day of anaerobic HIIT training, one day of aerobic low-intensity exercise and three days of bodyweight resistance training.

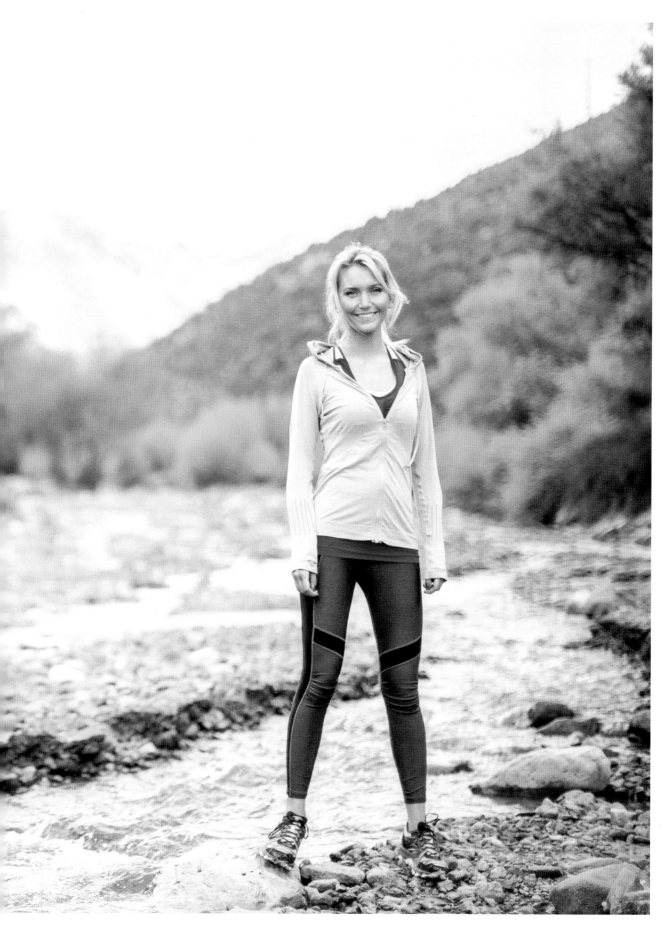

WARMING UP AND COOLING DOWN

I regularly see people dash out of the office, straight into the gym and start bench pressing massive weights without pausing to warm up. Almost as often, I see people run out of the gym at the end of their workout without properly cooling down. Choosing to ignore these crucial steps is not good for your fitness — and can be dangerous.

WHY WARM UP?

Warming up properly prepares the body for the main event and helps prevent injury. It's a 'starter' that fires up the central nervous system so that your muscles twitch quicker (see p.140), do their thing, and are fully 'switched on'. I like to think it's the same as warming up an F1 car to make sure the engine and tyres are in top condition before the big race! The best warm-ups are tailored to the types of demand you're about to put on your body.

WARMING UP FOR RESISTANCE TRAINING

The most effective way to warm up for resistance training is to think about the full exercise you're about to do and to introduce it gradually to your body, increasing the challenge in a progressive way. For example, if there's a big leg workout coming, the warm-up should specifically ensure your legs are prepared for it. Don't just dive directly into doing an Olympic squat with a loaded weight bar across your shoulders! Warm up with a few sets of bodyweight squats (that's just you and the squat) first, then add the bar, and then add weight to the bar slowly, so that your body knows what to expect and is ready to go for the real set at the top of your range. Bodyweight is always the best way to start.

WARMING UP FOR HIIT

As HIIT is a vigorously energetic form of cardio, it's well worth putting in a quick 'dynamic stretching' warm-up first, to mobilise the joints and make the body more supple ahead of the intense bursts. The low-down on forms of stretching is in the box on the opposite page.

STRETCH IT OUT!

There are two types of stretching:

DYNAMIC STRETCHING

This type is most relevant to weight-training and is usually a pre-workout 'stretching while moving' routine that includes lunges, walking lunges, reaching, power skipping, knee hugs and quad walks, among others.

STATIC STRETCHING

This type tends to be post-workout and is most relevant for bodyweight resistance training, such as the exercises in the three-week plan in Chapter 4. It is 'stretching while stationary' and is not about sweating, but, like the stretches on pages 148–154, aims to lengthen and relax the muscles. Static stretches are slow and constant. You should aim to hold each for up to 30 seconds, until you start to find them mildly uncomfortable. Try not to bounce while holding a static stretch, as bouncing can risk tearing muscle fibre.

WHY IS STRETCHING IMPORTANT?

What can stretching do for you? Plenty! Stretching helps you to:

▶ RETAIN MUSCLE BALANCE Stretching as part of your cool-down routine helps to prevent muscle imbalance that can lead to problems with your posture.
▶ REDUCE DOMS DOMS stands for 'delayed onset muscle soreness', otherwise known as that aching muscle pain you get a few days after working out – the thing that makes it hard to walk, sit down, use your arms... ! After a big workout your muscles will remain in a slightly contracted state. The best way to speed the recovery and avoid too much of the dreaded DOMS is to stretch a lot afterwards. It'll elongate and soften the muscle fibres, which will help re-condition you for your future training as well.
▶ GAIN FLEXIBILITY A good stretch will massively improve your range of motion – this means, for example, that with regular stretching you might be able to reach your toes if you bend over from standing with your legs straight, or perhaps even do the splits eventually!
▶ REDUCE THE RISK OF INJURY DRASTICALLY Because stretching improves flexibility and mobility, athletes who stretch properly are less likely to experience injury. Furthermore, regular stretching, alongside regular, appropriate exercise, will keep you mobile and less likely to suffer injury as your body matures.

In addition, regular stretching generally helps to keep your body in good condition. If you often spend long periods sitting at your desk, breaking only to get coffee, your muscles will tighten and weaken. Stretching out core parts of your body – the pelvis, hips, back, neck and shoulders – for just a few minutes every day helps to keep your body supple, ready for another day of hardcore chair-sitting!

WHY COOL DOWN?

Cooling down doesn't refer to your body temperature, but rather winding down your fired-up muscles. It is equally as important as warming up. If you don't cool down, your muscles will become increasingly tight, which can affect your future training as you won't enjoy the same range of motion, which in turn will impact your technique... which in turn means you're more likely to get injured. Cooling down is a key part of workout etiquette that everyone should add into their repertoire!

STATIC STRETCHING

The following static stretches (on pp.148–154) target all your major muscle groups (see pp.142–3). You can practise them all, in sequence, every day to keep your body in good condition, or you can practise specific stretches before or after working out, paying particular attention to the muscle groups you're targetting during that session. Hold each static stretch as directed, remember to stretch on both sides of your body to maintain balance, and also remember – don't bounce (see box, p.147)!

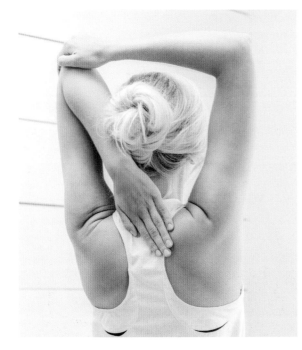

TRICEPS STRETCH Stand tall, feet firmly planted on the ground, shoulder-width apart. Bend your left arm and lift your left elbow towards the sky, tucking it towards your ear. Raise your right hand over your head and hold your left elbow. Apply gentle pressure with your right hand to guide the left arm back. You should feel the stretch along your left triceps muscle (at the back of your upper arm). Hold this stretch for 5 to 10 seconds, then repeat with the other arm. Repeat three times on each side.

'Regular stretching generally helps to keep your body in good condition.'

CHEST STRETCH Stand tall, feet planted firmly on the ground, shoulder-width apart. Interlock your hands behind your back, palms facing upwards towards the ceiling. Lift your chest and, keeping a straight back, pull your hands back and away from your body. You should feel the stretch across your chest. Hold for 10 to 20 seconds.

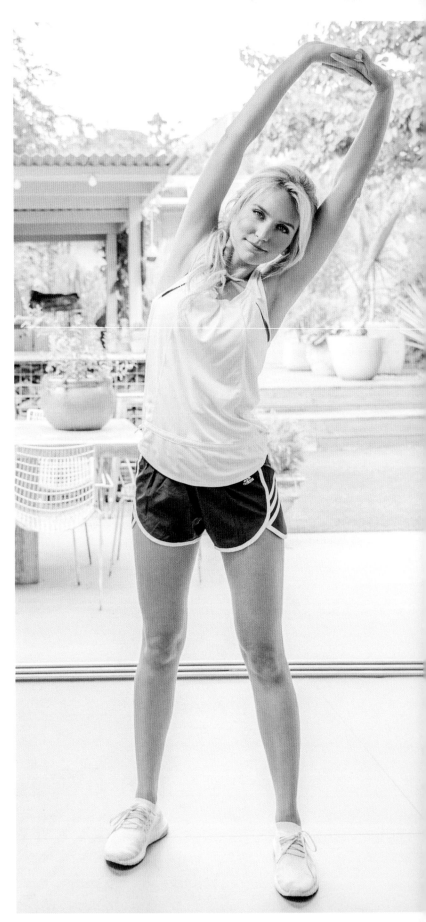

STANDING SIDE STRETCH

Stand tall, feet firmly planted on the ground, shoulder-width apart. Interlock your hands at waist height in front of you. Lift your hands towards the sky, turning your palms outwards so that they face up to the clouds. Lengthen and extend your body upwards. Hold the upright position for 5 to 10 seconds. Then, starting at the hip, slowly bend to the left as far as you can go, taking care to keep your whole body on the same plane (as if you're flat as a sheet of paper) – avoid twisting forwards at your hip. Hold the extent of the stretch for 5 to 10 seconds, then return slowly to the upright position and repeat on the right side. Repeat three times on each side.

STANDING QUAD STRETCH Stand facing a wall so that it is within arms reach (in case you need to hold on for balance). Keep your feet together, spine straight and your arms by your sides. Bend your left knee bringing your heel to your bottom, and gently push your hips forwards. Use your left hand to hold your left foot, feeling the stretch in your left quads (thigh muscles). Steady yourself with your right hand on the wall if you need to. Hold this stretch for 20 seconds. Release and repeat this time bending your right leg to stretch your right quads and using your left hand to steady yourself if you need to.

WALL CALF STRETCH (inset picture) This is a super-easy stretch! Face a wall, far enough away that your arms are bent at the elbows when you place both hands on it. Flex your left foot and step forwards so that your toes are touching the wall and your heel is on the floor. You should feel the stretch in your calf. After 10 to 30 seconds, swap legs. Alternatively, find a stair or curb and stand with your heels overhanging the top edge. One at a time, dip your heels to stretch your calves.

HAMSTRING STRETCH You can practise this stretch seated or standing. For the seated stretch (as in the picture), sit on the floor, back straight, legs straight out in front of you, knees pointing upwards. Pivoting forwards from your hips, gently reach forwards with your arms bringing your hands along your shins towards your feet. Go to where you feel comfortable and hold the stretch for 10 to 30 seconds. Remember this is not a competition, so just hold to the point where you feel the stretch, but it's not painful.

If the seated hamstring stretch isn't enough, try a standing stretch. Stand with your back to a wall, heels touching the wall behind you.

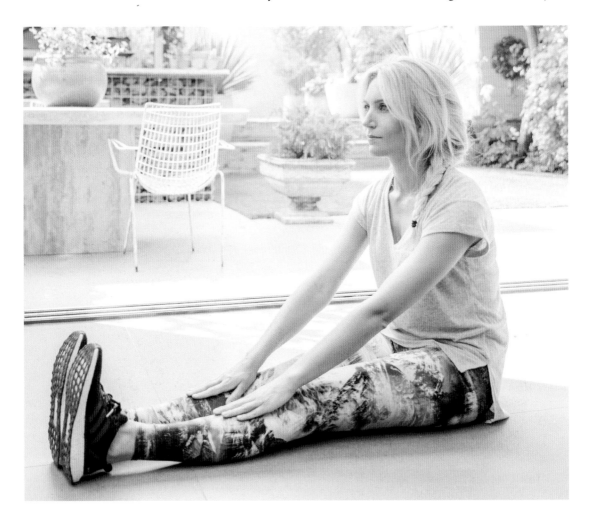

Bend forwards from your waist, pivoting at your hips, allowing your hands to stretch towards your feet.

SITTING GLUTE STRETCH Sit upright on the floor with both legs straight out in front of you. Bend your left leg, bringing your left foot over your right knee and putting it back on the floor on the right side of your right knee. Place your left hand on the floor behind you for support. Maintaining a straight back, use your right hand to pull your left leg towards your chest until you feel a stretch in your left glutes. Hold the stretch for 10 to 20 seconds, then swap legs. I like to do this a few times on each side.

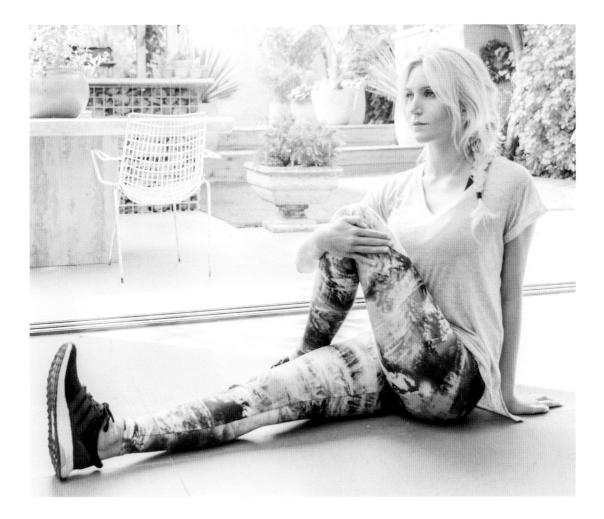

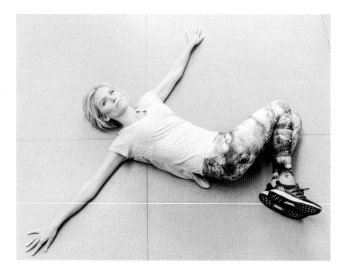

KNEE ROLLS Lie on your back, knees bent and feet flat on the floor. (You can place a pillow under your back for comfort, if you like.) Keep your legs together and open your arms wide. Relax your upper body. Slowly and in a controlled manner, roll your knees over to the left, allowing your pelvis to follow, but keeping both shoulders on the floor. Hold for 10 to 20 seconds, return to your starting position, then roll your knees to the right. Move only as far as feels comfortable, remembering that both your shoulders should stay planted on the floor. You should feel the stretch in your lower back.

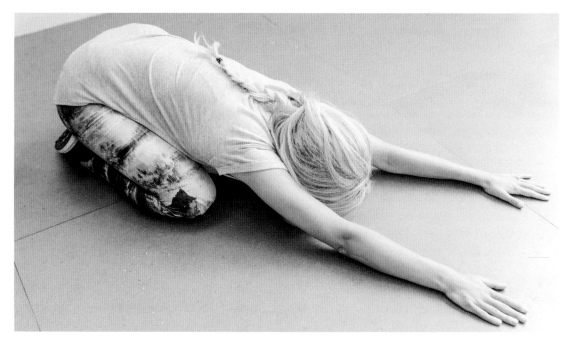

CHILD POSE Kneel on the floor (use a mat if you like) with your legs and knees together. Drop your bottom and sit back on your heels. Look straight ahead. Inhale, then exhale deeply and let your torso fold over onto your thighs until your forehead is resting on the floor in front of you. Extend your arms, resting your palms on the floor ahead. A yoga pose, this stretch is wonderful for gently extending your spine, neck and shoulders. Hold for as long as you feel comfortable.

MASSAGE IT OUT!

Sports massage is certainly not a cosmetic, chill-out treatment like you might find at a spa; it's an intense dose of focused, physical therapy administered by qualified sports massage professionals. If you've never had a sports massage, I strongly recommend you try! It can massively help prevent injury, relieve muscle pain (especially after training) and increase mobility. Massage helps improve circulation, increasing oxygen supply in the blood, and the flow of nutrients from the blood into the muscles and body tissues. It aids the body's detoxification process, helping to clear out metabolic waste as a result of exercise (such as lactic acid, the natural by-product of exercise that can cause stiffness and pain) and improve relaxation.

Of course, it's not always possible to go to a qualified sports therapist to receive these benefits. Here are ways to gain some of the benefits at home.

USE A FOAM ROLLER

While it may sound like some psychotropic drug at an Ibizan foam party, foam rollers are in fact a key physiotherapy tool. These little, soft cylinders can increase blood-flow, helping to flush out toxins and soften muscles for faster recovery. It's kind of like a DIY acupressure technique, or simply a nice massage. Using your own bodyweight against the roller, you manipulate your soft muscle tissue, supporting and massaging entire muscle groups while improving balance, stabilisation, flexibility and core strength.

Foam rollers come in different densities, from relatively soft foam to high density that feels less like foam and more like granite. When it comes to choosing what's right for you, I think the more accomplished, athletic and muscular the user, the denser the roller should be. Use the softest if you're new to exercise, working up to the hardest as you progress. Target your most tender areas, aiming to release the knots of overactivity. Frankly, doing this can border on painful – much in the same way that correct stretching feels mildly uncomfortable. Always distinguish between moderate discomfort and the pain that can lead to injury – your body will tell you the difference loud and clear, so stop if something hurts significantly.

USE A TENNIS BALL

Interesting idea! But, using a tennis ball is an awesome way to help neutralise muscular discomfort. For example, if I ever suffer from lower back pain, more often than not it's partly related to tight glutes. Tennis balls are the right treatment for this. To target my glutes, I'll 'sit' or lean against the ball on a wall, pressing it against my glutes to really work down beyond the superficial to the deep muscles. It's somewhat painful but, I think, better than anything else for getting to those stubborn knots in areas that require more precision than a foam roller can give. I find the tennis ball massage to be the most effective in the muscles of the back, bottom and hips. It's a focused pressure point that offers a superb release!

HIIT TRAINING

HIIT – or, to give it its full name, high-intensity interval training – is the godfather of all cardio and not for the faint-of-heart… literally. But it is a very effective and time-efficient exercise for anyone who struggles to fit a workout into a busy day. In the three-week plan in Chapter 4, you'll be doing one HIIT session a week.

MY HIIT

My personal favourite HIIT routine is to find a hill in the park, dispatch a bunch of burpees, runners and star jumps, and then sprint up the hill; Primrose Hill (Regent's Park) or Parliament Hill (Hampstead Heath) are two great local options for me, as they both deliver world-class views to really motivate me after struggling to the top. The sense of achievement when reaching the summit, standing atop the world looking out over London is pretty unbeatable. My advice is to find a place that inspires you come rain or shine, as you'll need to be there, come rain or shine!

HIIT IT HARD!

HIIT training involves alternating between intense bursts of activity and relatively relaxed action (known as the 'recovery period'), with the constant motion keeping your heart rate elevated. You set the level, but the main point is that during the 'on' period of your workout, you push yourself into that uncomfortable anaerobic zone (see p.144).

As always, it's important to listen to your body. If you're new to training or you haven't worked out for a while, you may find that your interval training needs to alternate between, for example, power walking and jogging. Others who are more comfortable with the technique will sprint and run. Finding your level and then slightly exceeding it is the whole point.

You can apply HIIT to any cardiovascular training – skipping, running, rowing, running up and down stairs – as long as you follow the same principle of high-energy 'bursts' alternating with more relaxed activity.

WHY HIIT?

Because 15 minutes is all you need – it's time efficient, burns more calories than traditional cardio in a smaller amount of time, maintains muscle while toasting fat, develops lung capacity, and stimulates the production of human growth hormone, which increases calorie burn even further! You don't even need a gym membership because you can practise HIIT pretty much anywhere, nor do you require any special equipment (just your body – and that's special enough already). Finally, if you're looking for a challenge, this heart-healthy session will push you to work at around 80- to 90-per-cent effort, leaving you really huffing and puffing.

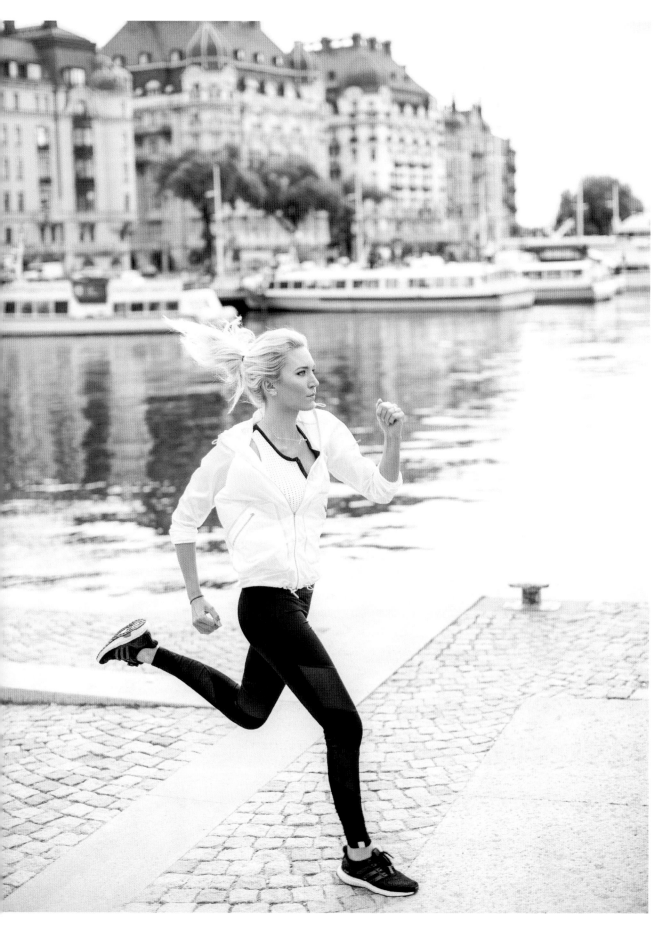

LOW-INTENSITY TRAINING

As much as I love HIIT training (see p.156), I strongly believe that all good training programmes need some low-intensity exercise added into the mix, and you'll be doing one low-intensity day a week as part of my three-week training plan in Chapter 4.

Low-intensity exercise is any exercise that raises the heart-rate, but, unlike HIIT, keeps activity at a steady, sustained level for a prolonged period of time. Low-intensity exercise is not an amble or a gentle stroll to the shops, but mid-pace (working at around 50 to 75 per cent of your maximum effort), steady cardiovascular training that you do continuously for 30 to 60 minutes.

As long as the exercise you choose is something you can sustain for the required amount of time, and at the same level, that's fine. Swim, cycle, row, or power walk (my favourite option; see box opposite) or hop on the cross-trainer or elliptical machine at the gym – just keep it slow and steady!

WHY DO IT?
As well as the very real benefits to your fitness – decreasing injury risk by being easier on the joints, increasing calorie burn, and stabilising blood sugar during and after exercise, among them – a day of low-intensity training will aid your body's recovery from your HIIT sessions and add variety into your routine to keep things interesting and stop you getting bored.

WHEN TO DO IT?
You can incorporate your low-intensity workout at any time during the day, but my preference is very early. If you can bear to get up an hour earlier (before breakfast) than you usually do that's ideal, as your glycogen stores (the way in which your body stores carbohydrate for energy) are generally depleted, which means the stored energy will be your body's major source of fuel rather than your brekkie!

POWER WALKING

My preference for low-intensity exercise is power walking, and it's what I've included in the plans in Chapter 4. It's an awesome fat burner and kind to your joints – which is great if you find running a challenge. You can do it indoors on a treadmill, outside in a beautiful setting, or indeed on your way to work, killing two birds with one stone. Switch on your favourite playlist, pop in your earphones and enjoy the breeze on your face; it can be a beautiful way to zone out!

Aim for a gentle but challenging incline and walk at around 6 km/h (roughly 3½ mph) or more for 30 to (ideally) 60 minutes – you can use a smartphone app to track your speed if that's helpful, or just make sure that your heart is pounding and you're slightly out of breath. Focus on standing tall – roll your shoulders back and down, use your arms to drive yourself forwards, keep your abdominals engaged and work your pelvic floor at the same time!

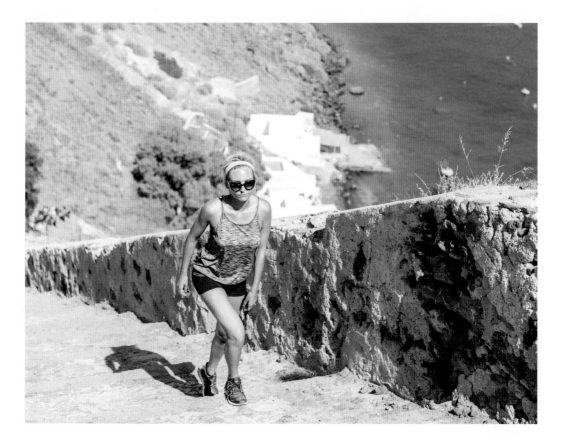

BODYWEIGHT RESISTANCE TRAINING

It won't have escaped your notice that gym memberships are expensive. In fact, fees can be so punchy that many workout fans find themselves priced out of the fitness game. But that doesn't have to mean that *fitness* should remain unachievable. That's why I advocate bodyweight resistance training, which makes the most of the awesome free tools you have available and that you carry around all the time. Rather than using a machine at the gym or an expensive piece of home equipment, it is *your own body* that provides the resistance. While you won't have all the facilities of a gym, you can have an effective and challenging workout from the comfort of your own home; a workout that you can do anywhere, any time, and that can be perfectly tailored to your fitness level.

Bodyweight exercises tend to mimic real-world, everyday movements – which generally means they're not too complicated! Take the mighty squat – an all-time favourite exercise of mine. To my mind the best way to execute the move is to imagine you're slowly sitting down onto a chair, and then reverse the motion back up. It really targets the legs and glutes and is also one of the top exercises for the core and abdominal midsection. If you're looking to achieve that illustrious six-pack, I'd argue that this bodyweight exercise is far better than thrashing out endless sit-ups.

For an extreme view of how effective the results of bodyweight training can be, search 'calisthenics' on YouTube, sort by view count and then sit back and enjoy an incredible array of urban street workouts that showcase amazing physiques and artistry.

The bodyweight exercises in my plan are less extreme, but still make use of several of your muscle groups. They also raise your heart rate, get you sweaty, and toast calories! Almost all the exercises progress every week, so that they become more challenging as your fitness improves. While always focusing on correct form, try to 'up' your repetitions in the time given in order to get the most out of your workout. If you can, try to do the exercises outdoors – being in nature always gives me a boost!

BODYWEIGHT 'CIRCUITS'

The type of bodyweight training in the plans is a blended combo of exercises. Just as with circuit training, you go from one 'station' to the next; only your own body provides the 'stations'. You'll need a timer, likely on your phone. Set it for 1 minute 'on' and 1 minute 'off'. During the 'on' phase, execute as many repetitions as possible. In the 'off' phase, rest, breathe deeply, lower your heart rate and prepare for the next exercise.

There are five exercises in total for each circuit workout and each circuit targets either upper-body, lower-body or full-body exercises, occurring on days 1, 3 and 5 of the plans respectively.

WILL I NEED EQUIPMENT?
None at all! You'll need just your own bodyweight and possibly a mat for comfort for the floor exercises – although grass would certainly do the job quite nicely! If you do have dumbbells at home and would like to include weights, please feel free to use them where appropriate – or use a big bag of sugar (that's the one time you'll find me advocating the use of refined sugar!).

BE PRECISE!
Focus on your technique, rather than number of repetitions. You're better off performing fewer repetitions well than doing lots badly, which can be ineffective and dangerous. Check your technique in the mirror and take your time to learn the exercises properly.

MIX IT UP!
Each week I introduce at least one variation and progression to the workout – a change in resistance or training frequency, for example – to ensure your training remains challenging. You want to avoid becoming a mouse on the wheel, doing the same thing over and over again – your body will adapt to the workout and the marginal benefit will be lower each time. Mixing things up and challenging yourself will neutralise the risk of reaching a benefit plateau.

STRETCH IT OUT!
After your workout your muscles will be in a seriously contracted state and need a proper stretching out. It's super-important not to overlook this so do use the stretches on pages 148–154.

ALWAYS REFUEL

Ideally, you should try to grab some replenishing food within an hour after your workout. If you're looking to lose weight it may seem counterintuitive, but this is prime time to eat, as your metabolism is running hot. The longer you leave it to replenish your body, the more likely you are to over-eat. Your body needs help to patch up the micro-tears exercising has made on your muscles, so getting a decent allotment of protein (a handful of nuts or some nut butter and veggie sticks are good options) immediately after your workout will help the healing process, so that your muscles can rebuild even stronger!

OTHER FORMS OF TRAINING

The three-week plan in this book is designed to kick-start your training; to make regular, daily exercise an essential part of your routine – something that you don't even think twice about. For that reason I've deliberately focused on a core group of simple exercises that will help you to make this fundamental change. But once you've nailed the basics, I'd recommend you try to expand your horizons! You might be comfortable in your routine, but there are three main reasons to embrace other – and perhaps more unusual – forms of training. Here they are:

1 THE GREAT OUTDOORS And I don't just mean going for a run around the neighbourhood, or doing your regular workout in the garden, I mean really getting out into nature and embracing the elements – come rain or shine!

2 THE SPICE OF LIFE Changing things up ensures you won't plateau. You need to surprise your body with unusual, challenging forms of exertion if it's going to make progress fitness-wise.

3 MAXIMUM FUN Don't underestimate this super-important consideration – a healthy, active life shouldn't be a prison sentence and mixing it up means you'll have more fun along the way!

Here's a small selection of my favourite forms of alternative exercise and reasons why I think they are so fantastic.

SAILING

One of my all-time favourite 'leisure' activities, sailing is hugely popular throughout Sweden owing to the country's extensive coastline. It's significantly more accessible than many people think (you can learn the basics on inland lakes) and, to be honest, not at all leisurely! You need physical strength and mental resolve, exemplary coordination and strong motor skills, as well as great core strength. You're leaning back much of the time, in a static hold that's keeping you from falling into the water; you're hoisting sails with your arms; and tensing your thighs much of the time. You're engaging all the little stabilising muscles that don't get out much, just to stay upright. It's a serious full-body workout, and – most importantly – loads of fun!

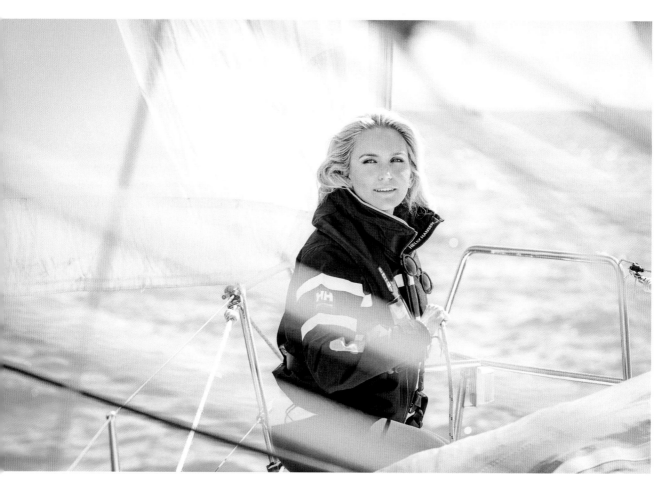

HIKING

Not to be confused with simply 'walking'! This is endurance cardio
that will burn a little under two-and-a-half times more calories
than an equivalent walk. A good hike usually involves getting
right out into the countryside, where you'll meet varied terrain,
altitudes, inclines, and weather conditions. You'll be able to beef
up your lower-body tone, build bone strength, develop your
stamina, work on your coordination – and, best of all, you can
take it at your own pace. While doing all this, you'll be breathing
in the freshest of air and seeing beautiful natural sights. Grab a
buddy and get to it!

SWIMMING

Competitive swimmers are some of the most physically fit athletes
on the planet. Their sport delivers an intense full-body workout
– all without feeling the discomfort of sweating! The broad range
of motion helps the joints to loosen up and become more flexible,
and the reduced gravity means it's practically impact-free, which
is great for those with joint pain. The water gives a constant level

of resistance, so that every kick or stroke is weighted, helping to develop muscle strength, as well as heart and lung strength from the intense aerobic activity. After a while, you settle into a leisurely autopilot rhythm, which is awesome for endorphin production.

HORSE RIDING

I grew up riding around a farm, so I can vouch that horse riding is a gruelling workout – but also truly exhilarating. Galloping with the wind licking at your face is a real adrenaline kick, and you'll be working your body in a most unfamiliar way. The inner thighs burn from clenching the horse's body, and you work the abdominals and obliques as a result of stabilising the body during a gallop. Your shoulders and arms are constantly working hard to grasp the reins. There's no slouching on this unstable pitch, and while it won't get you into 'bikini shape', riding will bring some proper strength gains – and it's a liberating, therapeutic activity that'll get you outdoors more often!

SKIING

Apart from being a great social occasion and a classic Nordic pursuit, skiing is essentially squatting for an extended period time, engaging all those same major muscle groups and reaping all the benefits. Controlling those alien planks attached to the rigid coffins on your feet takes fine adjustments, and uses muscles beyond those found in a squat – the calves and foot arches are surprisingly involved, too. You also need to stretch, as ski technique takes suppleness, and comes in handy when (sorry, if) you fall!

KETTLE BELLS

Kettle bells came from 18th-century Russia, where farmers weighed their crops against them. These days, they deliver a conveniently portable full-body workout that builds power and burns fat. Their handles distribute weight unevenly, which means you work on grip strength, core engagement, and coordination to wield them. That, in turn, develops muscles through the arms, shoulders and other stabiliser muscles, because they're inherently imbalanced, unlike a dumbbell. Best of all, they're cheap to buy, and you can take them to your local park for a change of scenery.

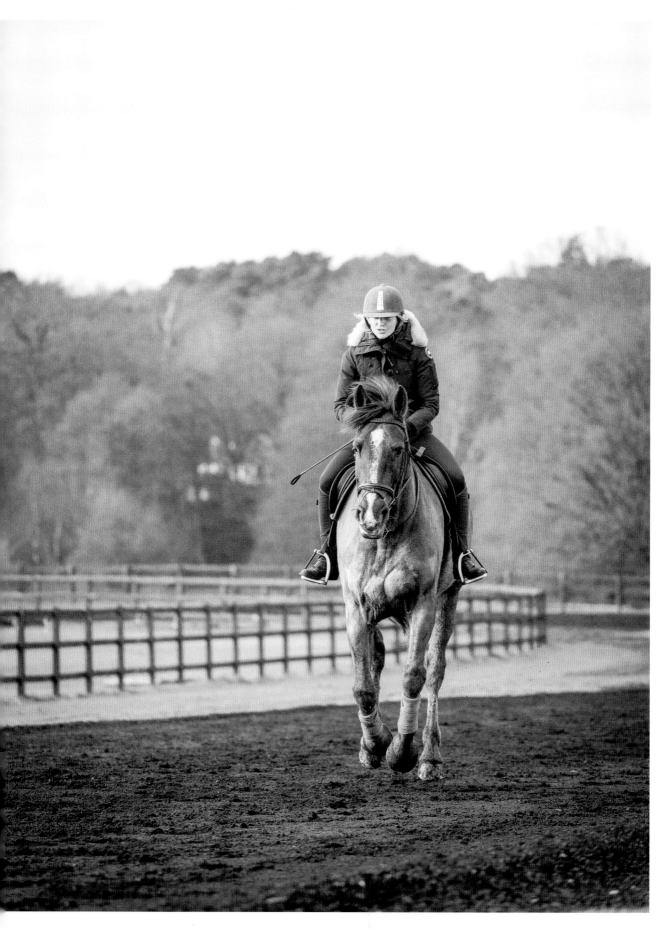

WHY WEIGHT TRAIN?

Modern exercise regimes seem increasingly eager to see us lift weights. Indeed, aesthetics aside, we generally accept that weight training is 'good', but do we really understand why? There are many physiological reasons why it is true that weight training is good for you, but I don't think we need necessarily preoccupy ourselves with the science. My experience tells me that weight training generally makes the body a little bit better at everything – speed, strength and endurance. Lifting weights is like sharpening a carving knife: you can still slice with a blunt knife, but when the knife is razor sharp, cutting is more efficient and the slices are more precise. A trained body is far more efficient and accurate in its movement and motion.

BOOSTING METABOLISM

Both during and after weight training, your body experiences a thermogenic effect: it generates heat, which burns calories. In fact, your muscular system is the largest metabolically active organ in your body and the effects play out even after your session has finished. The more muscle mass you have, the more efficient your metabolism will be; and, put simply, muscles burn fat!

When you start serious weight training, you may gain weight – but fear not. The reason is that muscle is denser than fat and so it weighs more. Rather than looking at the scales, think about your tone. A given weight in muscle occupies less space in your body than the same weight in fat – you'll look leaner, even if the scales appear to tell a different story. By lifting weights, you're creating micro-tearing in the muscle fibres, causing them to rebuild stronger when they repair. This action results in a more defined look to the musculature. It's about sculpting that body!

BUILDING STRONGER BONES

One of the main benefits of weight training is its positive effect on your bones. With age comes a totally normal decline in muscle mass and bone density, especially in women over the age of thirty. Weight (and strength) training has been shown to increase bone mass and decrease the risks of developing osteoporosis (weakening of the bones), leading to a skeleton that stays stronger for longer. Increasing the stress on bones – that is, forcing your bones to bear more weight than they are used to, through such exercise as weight lifting (but also running and other impact training) – encourages the growth of bone fibres, knitting your bone structure together more tightly and so improving bone density. Weight training is better for you than running, because it provides a mild impact on your bones that fortifies them but avoids the negative, jarring effects of the pounding that happens during footfall. There's no better way to gain the benefits than strength training with free weights, which applies the most direct and targeted stress impact to your bones without 'shocking' them.

MOVE, THEN LIFT

Before you think about weight training, you need to make sure you're moving. Back in the day we moved a lot: we grew our fresh produce, so we spent time planting and harvesting; we did manual jobs to earn a living; we always hung out the washing (who thought we'd one day just turn a switch on a tumble dryer!); we walked rather than tapping for an Uber to come to find us – and so on. Now, so many of us sit at desks in front of screens for 12 hours a day – lots of people I know barely walk further than the water cooler in a whole day at the office.

It's a cliché but, if you can, take the stairs instead of the lift. Run up the escalators on the subway. At the office, walk about while on your phone call. Go for a 10-minute walk at lunchtime or dash out to a fitness class. When you get home, stretch while you're watching TV. If you can train – in whatever form that training might present itself – do it! The more you move, the better for your body. Once you get into the mindset that movement can become part of your daily life – even your modern daily life – you'll appreciate how movement makes you feel better, every day.

Then, supplement your movement with weight training (remember, sharpen the knife!). Sitting for hours weakens the gluteus muscles (in your bottom) and increases your susceptibility to lower back problems, along with other aches and pains. Some muscles will naturally become tighter and weaker just because we sit for too long. The good news is regular moving combined with weight training helps arm us with strong, resilient bodies to fend off these ailments!

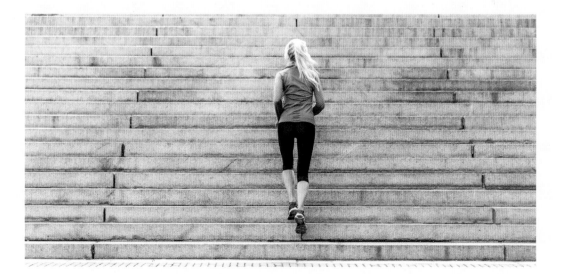

GOOD BALANCE, STRONG JOINTS AND A HEALTHY HEART

Not only does weight training improve bone density (see p.166), but the improved muscle power that comes from weight training strengthens your core and can even out imbalances in the sides of your body (because you focus on developing muscles on each side specifically). The results are that your joints become stronger and you achieve better posture and balance.

Another interesting benefit of weight training is that it develops the muscles around the heart, therefore improving the strength of your heart. It helps to lower resting blood pressure slightly, too.

All of this is great for ageing – better posture and balance means reduced risk of falls, and a heart that pumps healthily will be better placed to serve you well into your twilight years.

Improving bone density through weight training is a relatively slow process, but it is a serious investment into your health pension.

'WILL I GET BULKY?'

If I had ten Swedish *krona* for every time a girl asked me this! Gaining significant amounts of muscle takes serious hard work and dedication – even for men, whose testosterone levels (testosterone is a steroid hormone) are much higher than women's anyway. It's way more difficult for girls to pile on the muscular bulk. Those few women you may see in the gym who look vast have most likely worked incredibly long and hard to attain that very specific bodyshape! In short, there's no need to worry about 'bulking up'. The chances of waking up one morning splitting your blouse sleeves because you lifted heavy weights the night before are… zero!

However, if you *are* worried about gaining size, there are certain muscle groups (and therefore certain exercises) that you might de-emphasise. The trapezius (in the neck and surrounding area;

see p.142) is a good example – a thick neck is a look most women don't care to develop. Likewise, few mademoiselles want comically pronounced quadriceps (thigh muscles). But, what woman doesn't want a perky, round, firm butt – which, by the way, is the gift you get from almighty squats and thunderous dead lifts! Or toned arms and defined shoulders? So start benching, or keep lifting heavier.

TOP TIPS FOR GETTING STARTED

1 WARM UP FIRST That doesn't mean a 20-minute run, it simply means to warm up the body with exercises that mimic the workout ahead. For example, if you're about to do a massive leg session, do some squats and lunges; or you could do some burpees, jumping jacks and so on. Try to include some dynamic stretches, too (there's more on stretches on pages 148–154).

2 GO LARGE, THEN GO SMALL Organise your weights session so that you start lifting using larger muscle groups first and finish off with exercises that require more precise muscle work. For example, a weighted pull-up requires several muscles to work together to muster the required strength. If you try to do pull-ups after, say, tiring your arms out with targetted triceps' weight exercises you're less likely to be able to perform the pull-ups effectively.

3 START WITH COMPLEX EXERCISES Do more complicated exercises first. So, if you're doing a leg workout, for example, dispatch the deadlifts early on, as they require way more mental focus, as well as more difficult technique and greater overall strength. If you leave something that requires such mental and physical acuity to the end, when you're both mentally and physically tired already, you won't perform them as well, meaning the benefits are fewer and you're at greater risk of injury.

4 WARM DOWN LAST! Finish with a minimum of 10 minutes of static stretching (see pp.148–154) remembering that this is an important part of any workout to allow your muscles to readjust slowly and to minimise the injury risk and the dreaded DOMS.

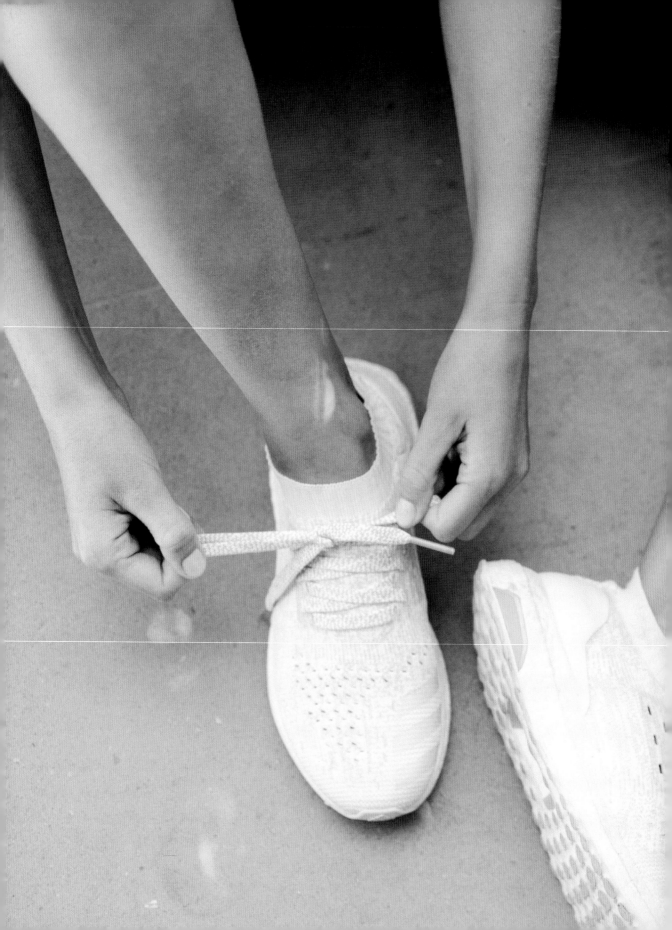

CHAPTER 4

THE Three-week Training Plan

'Day-by-day guidance on how to eat, how to be mindful, and how to use your body to promote wellness.'

THE POWER OF THREE

Welcome to my three-week training plan! Before you start, though, I want to recap on something that is really important to me – the principle that underpins everything this book is about.

No, it isn't bulging biceps! This plan doesn't pretend to be a 'bikini body' three-week plan. Nor does it masquerade as a 'six-pack-quick-fix' scheme. Throughout the book, I've mooted the idea of sustainability – which is the polar opposite of any drastic, short-term fitness diversion that would see you operate under a calorie deficit, while crushing it in the gym for two or more hours a day. The notion of a 'quick fix' sells a lot of magazines each year, often around May before the summer holidays. It's a seasonal panic advocating an approach that flusters me: it's unattainable, unrealistic and, ultimately, unhealthy. With a supposed quick fix, you're more likely to end up fatigued, miserable, having to abandon all social life, and resenting what had once been presented as 'good for you'.

Rather, over the following pages I'll give you day-by-day guidance on how to eat, how to be mindful and how to use your body to promote wellness. I hope that over the course of three weeks, you'll see that being 'Scandi fit' isn't about slavishly following a nutritional regime or pumping it in the gym, but about gently and sustainably adapting your lifestyle so that eating well, thinking clearly, and looking after your physical body become part of everyday life, always.

The principle of the three-week plan is like one of those fitness aphorisms that 'it takes three weeks to form a good habit or kick a bad one'. The notion of 'bad habits', though, suggests that we need to extinguish elements of ourselves. In this three-week plan, however, it's not about scaling back, but about introducing more: more delicious recipes, more variation in your diet and exercise, more healthy snacks. The plan provides different forms of exercise that build in elements of strength training, HIIT, low-intensity cardiovascular training, and flexibility. It's a realistic approach, and one for which the ultimate target is 'healthy for life'.

On every day of the plan you'll find:

- A meal-by-meal menu: this uses the recipes in the book to make sure that every day your diet is nutritionally balanced, satisfying, delicious and, therefore, in all ways good for you. On the first day of each week, the plan provides a 'meat-free Monday' – a day with no meat at all.
- A mindfulness tip: this might be something to think about or to do, but is intended to help you bring focus and thoughtfulness into your life in natural, everyday ways.
- A physical sequence or fitness idea to help you use your body so that it stays balanced and toned. Over the three weeks, the bodyweight resistance plans work your upper body, lower body and full body, in turn. Some days are rest days – these are important, too. Remember that exertion every day is not a good thing – your body needs to rest and recover.

Over the three weeks, the fitness sequences in each week will get slightly harder, pushing you slightly further so that your practice continues to motivate you. As you progress through the programme, the exercises will get easier to do. In this case, and if you want to keep progressing, try adding repetitions. Do what feels comfortable, achievable and good. And, most of all, enjoy!

A PROGRAMME FOR EVERYONE

The whole training programme is designed to rely exclusively upon your body weight. Sounds easy? Not in the slightest! You can achieve exceptional results with nothing more than your own mass, which is the whole theory underpinning calisthenics. When I've suggested it, you can add weight, but this is by no means a requirement. Perhaps this is your first week training almost every day in a long time, or perhaps you're a regular gym-goer. Each workout is designed to be challenging for everyone regardless of fitness level. You are in control: adjust each workout according to your experience and capability.

WEEK 1

'You don't have to be great to start, but you have to start to be great.' ZIG ZIGLAR (1926–2012), US MOTIVATIONAL SPEAKER AND AUTHOR

That's one of my favourite quotations; it reminds us that everybody, regardless of age, gender or experience, must start somewhere. Even Olympic legend Usain Bolt didn't spring forth from the womb in 9.58 seconds – he, too, had to crawl before he could run very, very fast. Welcome to your first week of my plan – it's a time to really listen to your body, to push yourself more than you may have ever done before, and to pat yourself on the back at the end of every session. Whether you're trying something new or getting back into it, you're doing great just by having set your mind to it. That mental resolve counts for a lot in the world of fitness! This week you'll be dispatching HIIT training, low-intensity training, body-weight exercises, and stretching sessions. You'll be experiencing a bunch of different ways to challenge your body. At times it will definitely feel tough – nothing worth having comes easily – but just remember that quotation. I promise you, the changes you make now, you'll thank yourself for in three weeks, two months, a year's time – and beyond. You'll quickly notice that you have more energy, you sleep better, you wake up feeling refreshed and you feel happier!

DAY 1

DAY 1: NUTRITION PLAN

BREAKFAST:	▶ Wake-me-up (p.134), then Max muesli (p.56)
MID-MORNING SNACK:	▶ Energy balls (p.126)
LUNCH:	▶ Rainbow salad with roasted spiced almonds (p.77)
MID-AFTERNOON SNACK:	▶ 1 apple
DINNER:	▶ Wild mushroom & spelt risotto (p.103)

DAY 1: MINDFULNESS PLAN

HYDRATE, HYDRATE, HYDRATE

Your mind and your body need water. I recommend you drink 200–250ml of 'good fluids' (see p.41) each hour. Remember my tip: grab a 1-litre bottle and a marker pen. Mark 200ml increments on the side of the bottle, and allocate 8am to the first line, 9am to the next line, then 10am and so on all the way to the bottom of the bottle. Then, use your lines to check you're drinking enough as you go about your day.

DAY 1: BODYWEIGHT RESISTANCE

1 WALKING LUNGE WITH REAR LEG RAISE

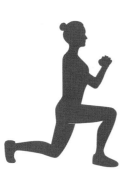 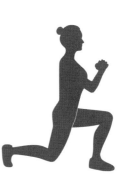

1 Stand tall, feet hip-width apart, relax your shoulders and look straight ahead. Engage your core by pulling your navel towards your spine. Step forwards with your right leg, dropping your hips to bend your knees until each leg forms a right angle. Take care not to let your right knee extend over your right toes, and don't let your left knee drop to the ground.

2 Pause for 1–2 seconds, then push off your right heel, and as you straighten up, raise your left leg up with the sole of your left foot pointing towards the sky and keeping your left leg as straight as possible. You should feel the effort in your glutes as you push up.

3 In one motion, as you reach the top of the raise, bring your left leg forwards past your right to lunge forwards with your left leg in front. Drop your hips into the lunge, pause, then raise your right leg as you come up again. Repeat, alternating left and right legs for 1 minute.

2 STATIC SQUAT

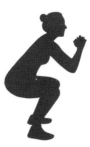

1 Stand tall and plant your feet shoulder-width apart, relax your shoulders and look straight ahead. Point your feet forwards. Link your fingers in front of your chest, bending your arms at your elbows.

2 Bending at the knees, lower yourself towards the floor, keeping your back straight, your abs engaged and your lower back as neutral as possible. Dig your heels into the floor to anchor yourself as you lower.

3 Push your hips backwards until your thighs are parallel to the floor. Avoid allowing your knees to extend beyond your toes. Hold the squat for 1 minute, or for as long as possible, feeling the effort in your quads. When you're ready, straighten your knees and come back up to standing.

3 GLUTE BRIDGE

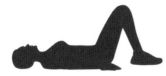 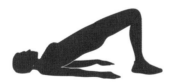 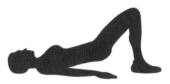

1 Lie on the floor (I recommend a mat for comfort), knees bent, feet flat on the floor, hip-width apart. Push your lower back into the floor to make sure your back isn't arched. Place your arms, palms down, by your sides.

2 Squeeze your glutes together, then using these gluteus muscles, lift your lower body off the floor pushing down through your feet. Ensure you keep your hips nice and square throughout.

3 When you've raised yourself as far as possible, pause and slowly and with control lower towards the floor again, ideally letting your bottom hover just above the floor rather than touching the floor. Go straight into the next repetition. Repeat the raise and lower for 1 minute.

4 GLUTE KICKBACK (1)

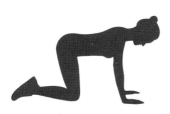

1 Start on the floor on all fours (use a mat for comfort). Position your hands roughly shoulder-width apart, directly under your shoulders, and ensure your knees are directly under your hips.

2 Engage your abdominals by pulling your navel towards your spine. Keeping your right leg bent at the knee, extend the leg behind you so that your right thigh is in line with your body and parallel to the floor, with the sole of your foot pointing towards the ceiling.

3 Contract your glutes, and keeping your right knee bent, lift your foot as high as possible. Then, slowly and with control, lower your knee towards the floor again. Tap your toes gently on the floor, then raise up again. Raise and lower for 1 minute, then repeat on your left leg.

5 SINGLE LEG DEADLIFT

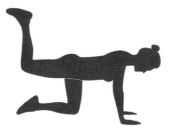

1 Stand tall, feet hip-width apart and well anchored. Transfer your weight to your right leg, ever-so-slightly bending your right knee (that is, not locked-out and totally straight). Raise your left foot a little off the ground. Engage your abs by pulling your navel towards your spine, and find your balance.

2 Pivot forwards at the hips, extending your left leg behind you. Keep your core engaged; avoid curving your back or hunching your shoulders. Slowly, with control lower your body and raise your left leg until it is parallel to the floor. Aim to create a T-shape with your legs and body. Allow your arms to hang down.

3 Slowly and with control, return to the starting position. Aim to dispatch 1 minute of continuous repetitions, extending and pivoting and returning to the start. Then, swap legs and repeat for a further 1 minute, standing on your left leg and extending your right leg behind you.

DAY 2

DAY 2: NUTRITION PLAN

BREAKFAST:	▶ Rocket fuel (p.131), then Apple & date mixed grain porridge (p.57)
MID-MORNING SNACK:	▶ Kale chips with za'atar (p.123)
LUNCH:	▶ Simple salad with crayfish & citrus dressing (p.72)
MID-AFTERNOON SNACK:	▶ 1 pear
DINNER:	▶ Marinated chicken with butternut squash & ginger mash (p.88)

DAY 2: MINDFULNESS PLAN

SWITCH IT OFF

Don't forget to turn off your electronics a good hour before your bedtime. TVs, computers, tablets, and mobile phones – anything that emits blue light – disrupt the balance of your body's natural sleep chemicals and makes it harder to get to sleep.

DAY 2: LOW-INTENSITY POWER WALK

Today is your first power-walking day (see pp.158–9)! 'Walking' probably doesn't sound particularly taxing, and you might even think 'Hmm… that sounds like a pointless stroll in the park… no benefit for me there.' Beat down the grumpy cynic within! It's not supposed to be quite that relaxed! The 'power' part is the clue that you are still supposed to go for it (remembering to work at 50 to 75 per cent of what you might consider maximum exertion). Nevertheless, power walking is very much a lower-intensity form of exercise (lower than HIIT, for example) that's soft on the joints and easier on the lungs! Aim to spend 1 hour power walking today – you'll burn 300 to 400 calories during that time, depending upon how hard you push it. All the time you'll be operating in the more comfortable 'aerobic zone' (see p.144), enjoying a surplus of oxygen, enabling your body to break down fat stores super efficiently. So, get up a little earlier, pop on your walking shoes, and get out there! Keep the pace quick, the arms swinging (to propel you onwards), and the music loud.

DAY 3

DAY 3: NUTRITION PLAN

BREAKFAST:	▶ Super-vit (p.131), then Eggs from the 'forest' (p.63)
MID-MORNING SNACK:	▶ On-the-go power bar (p.125)
LUNCH:	▶ Baked sweet potato with curried apple slaw (p.81)
MID-AFTERNOON SNACK:	▶ ½ papaya
DINNER:	▶ Prawn, anchovy & greens pasta (p.99)

DAY 3: MINDFULNESS PLAN

ZONE OUT

Find a quiet place to sit for 5 to 15 minutes. Make yourself comfortable, perhaps with your legs crossed, or even in the half-lotus meditation pose. Shut out all sound from your consciousness, close your eyes and focus on an imaginary point just behind your eyes... gently escape from the world.

DAY 3: BODYWEIGHT RESISTANCE

1 BEAR CRAWLS

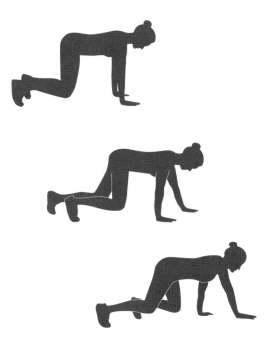

1 Start on the floor on all fours (use a mat for comfort), with your hands directly underneath your shoulders and your knees beneath your hips.

2 Push up onto your toes, raising your knees off the floor, but keeping them bent so that your back is completely straight and parallel to the ground (no arching or slouching). Engage your abs, by pulling your navel in towards your spine. Move forwards in a slow and controlled motion, starting with left arm and right leg forwards.

3 Then, switch to right arm, left leg, so that you're moving like a bear. At no point should your knees touch the floor, but roaring is optional. Move like this for 1 minute.

2 HALF PUSH-UP

3 ALTERNATING SUPERMAN

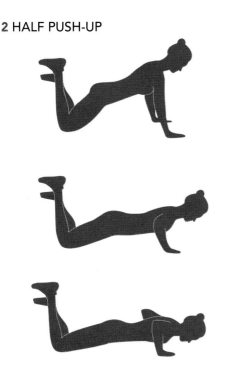

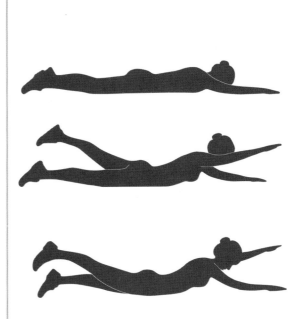

1 Lie face down on the floor. Place your hands to the sides of and in line with your shoulders, in a wide grip. Cross your ankles, raise your feet and, keeping your knees on the floor, push up with your arms so that you form a straight, diagonal line from the top of your head to your knees. Take care not to let your bottom sag.

2 Bending your elbows, inhale and slowly and with control, lower yourself downwards towards the floor.

3 Don't let your chest touch the floor, then once you are at the lowest point, exhale and press into your hands and straighten your elbows again, squeezing your chest and raising your upper body back up to the starting position. After a brief pause at the top, lower yourself downwards again for as many repetitions as you can manage in 1 minute.

1 Lie face down on the floor (use a mat for comfort). Extend your arms in front of your head and lengthen your legs behind you, the soles of your feet pointing towards the ceiling. Let both legs rest on the floor.

2 Lift your head so that your nose is hovering just above the floor, then simultaneously, raise your right arm and left leg off the floor, as if imitating the great Clark Kent himself (although not when he's in the office)! Hold the lift for 3–5 seconds.

3 Lower your right arm and left leg to the floor, then swap so that you raise your left arm and right leg. Hold again, then release. Keep alternating for 1 minute (or until you just can't fly anymore).

4 TRICEPS DIPS

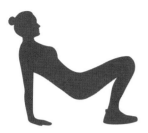

1 Sit upright on the floor with your back straight, knees bent with your feet flat on the floor and arms by your sides. Press your palms into the floor, straighten your arms and raise your bottom off the floor. Adjust the position of your feet, extending your legs a little if you need to, so that you get a good lift off the floor.

2 Using your feet to anchor yourself, push as high as you can go – leave a slight bend at your elbows so that they don't lock tight.

3 Keeping your elbows tucked in to your sides, slowly and with control bend your arms to lower your bottom towards the floor again, but without touching it to the floor. At the lowest part of the movement, slowly and with control push yourself back up to the starting position. Repeat the lowering and raising for 1 minute.

5 UPPER BACK BLASTER

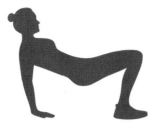

1 Lie face down on a mat on the floor, tuck your toes under and raise yourself onto your hands to put yourself into a plank position. Ensure you have a straight spine and you fire up your abdominals by drawing your navel in towards your spine. Relax your shoulders and neck muscles such that they're not bunched up towards your ears. You need a soft and neutral posture.

2 Slowly squeeze your shoulder blades together as hard and as much as you can without pain. Imagine you're squeezing something long and thin, like a stick, between your shoulder blades and trying to hold it there. Hold for 2–3 seconds, keeping your core strong and your body aligned throughout.

3 Release and return to your starting position, softening the posture once more. Repeat the squeeze, hold and release sequence for 1 minute. (Note: if you find this hard to do in the full plank, you can try it supporting yourself on your elbows, rather than your hands, in a low plank position.)

DAY 4

DAY 4: NUTRITION PLAN

BREAKFAST:	▶ Purple vitality (p.132), then Max muesli (p.56)
MID-MORNING SNACK:	▶ Savoury egg muffin (p.128)
LUNCH:	▶ Asian broth with chicken & mint (p.67)
MID-AFTERNOON SNACK:	▶ 2 celery sticks
DINNER:	▶ Herrings in oatmeal with rémoulade (p.94)

DAY 4: MINDFULNESS PLAN

SIT AT THE TABLE

Free time can feel so limited that we often try to do lots of things at once, rather than savouring every single thing for what it is. Tonight, there's no eating your food while sitting in front of the TV and catching up on your favourite drama. Instead, sit at the table to eat. Chew slowly and enjoy each mouthful, focusing on the textures and flavours of the food. Life shouldn't be a rush, and that means nor should dinner!

DAY 4: HIIT PLAN

Welcome to our first HIIT day – you're going to power out some bursts of highly energetic activity, followed by low-intensity recovery. Remember, it's all about getting the heart pumping! Today, jump on your bike and get into the great outdoors. Or, if that's not feasible, get on an exercise bike in the gym. Cycling is an awesome tool to help in your HIIT training, and it's gentle on your joints, too. You're going to mix it up: there will be some periods of gentle cycling interspersed with intervals of high-burst energy. The formula I opt for is: 1 minute of faster-paced activity, followed by a more relaxed, recovery pace of slow cycling, for 2 minutes. The total time for this alternating pattern should be 12 minutes, enabling you to power out four cycles of 1-minute-on-2-minutes-off. It might not sound like a lot of time, but this 'dirty dozen', so to speak, will have you in stitches (and not of laughter!).

DAY 5

DAY 5: NUTRITION PLAN

BREAKFAST:	▶ Vitamin-C bomb (p.134); Baked avocado with egg & trout tartare (p.60)
MID-MORNING SNACK:	▶ Energy balls (p.126)
LUNCH:	▶ Broad bean, mint & ricotta smörgås (p.78)
MID-AFTERNOON SNACK:	▶ 1 orange
DINNER:	▶ Seafood & fennel tagine with saffron aioli (p.96)

DAY 5: MINDFULNESS PLAN

RECHARGE WITH GREEN TEA

When you're looking for that 'comforting moment' (perhaps in the form of a sweet biscuit and/or hot chocolate), be mindful. Rather than succumbing to your natural impulse for a quick-fix sweetener, opt for something healthier, but no less comforting. A green tea and a few sweet berries on the side should do the trick!

DAY 5: BODYWEIGHT RESISTANCE

1 WALKING PLANK

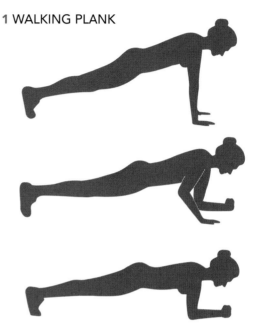

1 Put yourself into a full plank position – feet hip-width apart, toes tucked under, raised up on your straightened (but not locked) elbows, spine in alignment. Engage your abs. Make sure you form a straight line from the top of your head to your heels, and that your bottom isn't sagging or too high.

2 Slowly and with control release your left arm to plant your left forearm on the floor. Your body will tilt to the left, but keep your back straight!

3 Lower onto your right elbow, so that you are flat again. Then, slowly and with control, push into the floor with your right forearm and push up on your left so that you return your left hand into its original position, raising your left side. Follow with your right. Repeat the cycle (down, down; up, up) for 1 minute.

2 BURPEES

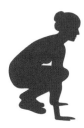

1 Stand straight with your feet hip-width apart and arms by your sides. Pull your navel in towards your spine to engage your abs.

2 Drop your hands to the floor, planting them slightly wider than shoulder-width apart just in front of you and jump back your feet, toes tucked under, so that you form a full plank position.

3 Engage your core and jump your feet forwards towards your hands as far as you can, then with one continuous movement spring back to your starting position. Repeat the sequence continuously for 1 minute.

3 MOUNTAIN CLIMBER

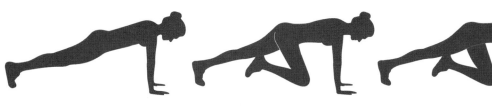

1 Begin by putting yourself into a full press-up position – feet hip-width apart, toes tucked under, raised up on your straightened (but not locked) elbows, spine in perfect alignment and shoulders over your wrists. Engage your abs by pulling your navel in towards your spine.

2 Bring your right knee forwards towards your right arm and touch the tops of your right toes to the floor. In a continuous 'running' movement, return your right leg back to the starting position.

3 As you do so, bring your left knee forwards towards your left arm, touching the tops of your left toes to the ground. How far forwards you can touch will depend on your flexibility. Go as far as you can, maintaining a straight spine throughout (don't raise your bottom). Keep the tempo high, alternating legs in and out as if two pistons are firing alternately. Continue for 1 minute, or until you have to stop.

4 TURKISH GET-UPS (BEGINNER)

1 Lie on your back on the floor (use a mat), legs out in front of you, arms by your sides. Take care not to arch your back. Lift your left arm directly up above you, fingers to the sky. Bend your left knee, placing your right heel close to your bottom. Move your left arm away from your body slightly. 'Lengthen' through your body.

2 Drive your weight through your left heel and push up onto your right elbow. Keep your chest up and out, stopping it from caving in as you lift your left side away from the floor. Look at your raised hand. Push your right hand into the floor.

3 With a straight spine come up to an almost-seated position. Then with control, unwind to lower yourself to the floor again, keeping your left hand in the air throughout. Repeat the sequence on your left side for 1 minute, then do it all again with your right arm raised and right knee bent, using your left arm for support.

5 BICYCLE KICKS

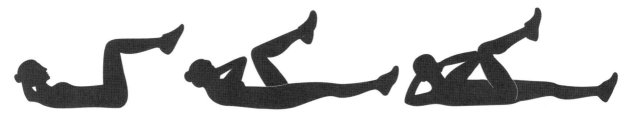

1 Sit on your bottom on the floor, legs out in front of you (use a mat for comfort), arms bent at the elbows and hands on either side of your head. Lean back, keeping your head raised, engage your abdominals and raise your legs off the floor, bending them at the knees and so that your thighs are perpendicular to the floor. Keep your ankles soft.

2 From the hip, bring your left knee towards your chest. Your right leg should extend but remain off the floor. At the same time, reach your right elbow to touch your left knee as it comes towards your chest. Take care not to pull on your head – just rest your fingers on the sides of your head and use your abdominals to create the reach.

3 Return to the starting position and immediately bring your right knee up to your chest and reach towards it with your left elbow. Return to the starting position. Continue to alternate left knee to right elbow and right knee to left elbow, keeping your legs raised from the floor, for 1 minute. Try to keep a good pace throughout.

DAY 6

DAY 6: NUTRITION PLAN

BREAKFAST:	▶ Immune Booster (p.135), then Tofu & spring onion pancakes (p.61)
MID-MORNING SNACK:	▶ Roasted spiced almonds (p.122)
LUNCH:	▶ Coconut, lentil & cardamom soup (p.68)
MID-AFTERNOON SNACK:	▶ Handful of blackberries
DINNER:	▶ Warm salad of roasted salmon, fennel & baby new potatoes (p.93)

DAY 6: MINDFULNESS PLAN

SIT UP STRAIGHT

Here's a good habit that will make you feel taller, brighter and more alert without an ab-churning plank in sight! Today, every time you stand or sit still, focus on your posture. Is your spine straight (no slouching)? Are your feet planted firmly on the floor? Are your shoulders aligned? If you're sitting at a computer, are your wrists and hands supported and is your screen directly in front of your face, so that your neck is straight? Simple care for your posture helps to ease the cumulative stress on your body.

DAY 6 AND 7: REST DAYS

Days 6 and 7 are your rest days – no HIIT or bodyweight resistance, or even low-intensity exercise to do! However, stretching out your body any day of the week is always good for you. So, if you feel like it, wake up on these days and practise your Sun Salutation (see pp.28–32 for full explanation) and in the process give your body a good stretch out for the day ahead. Begin in Mountain Pose, and then follow the sequence shown on the right, reversing it once you get to the end.

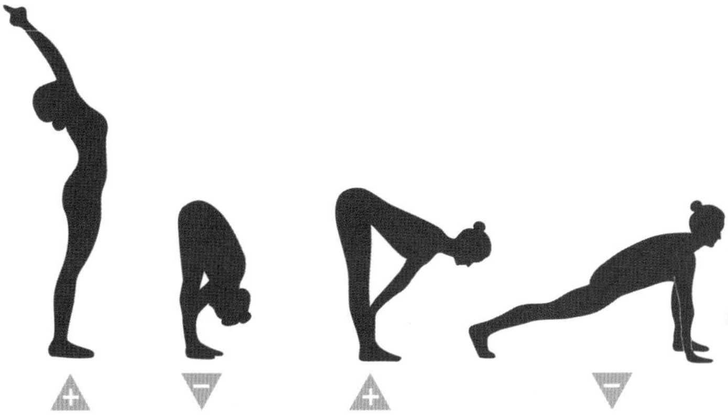

DAY 7

DAY 7: NUTRITION PLAN

BREAKFAST:	▶ Energiser (p.132), then Sundae for Sunday (p.58)
MID-MORNING SNACK:	▶ 1 pear
LUNCH:	▶ Roasted aubergine & sundried tomato salad (p.80)
MID-AFTERNOON SNACK:	▶ Three-nut butter (p.124) with fruit or on toast
DINNER:	▶ Tuna burger with fresh pickle (p.91)

DAY 7: MINDFULNESS PLAN

GET CREATIVE

Once in a while, starting today, sit down and just draw or paint, even if you're not that artistic. The practice of mindfulness is said to boost creative thinking. Mindfulness makes you more aware of all that's around you, which means you're more able to draw inspiration from your surroundings! Even simple doodling is amazingly therapeutic!

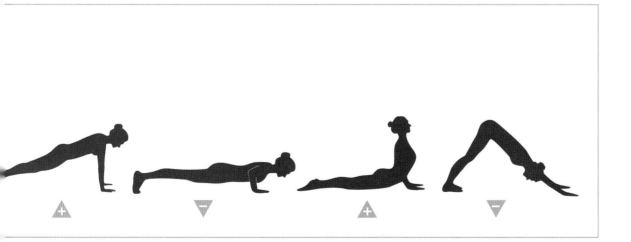

WEEK 2

'Weakness is the body getting stronger.'

ANONYMOUS

Great work – by now you've entered the second week of the readiness plan! Your body may feel a little sore here and there (don't forget to warm up, stretch, and cool down; see p.147). That physical weakness you might be feeling is totally normal, and is simply your body getting stronger. Your body is constantly in recovery mode, and to challenge it a little more (now that it's Week 2), we're going to step up the load we place on it. I've curated a measured increase in difficulty this week, specifically so that it places the right amount of extra strain on your musculoskeletal and aerobic/anaerobic systems. The exercises will become a little more intense, the duration slightly longer, and the HIIT more taxing. But your body should respond by releasing lots more of those happy chemicals! You'll feel more tired in the evenings ready to indulge in a night of restorative sleep, then to hit it hard all over again the following day! Let's get straight down to business…

DAY 1

DAY 1: NUTRITION PLAN

BREAKFAST:	▶ Wake-me-up (p.134), then Soufflé omelette with asparagus & walnuts (p.64)
MID-MORNING SNACK:	▶ Roasted spiced almonds (p.122)
LUNCH:	▶ Mini chickpea burgers with tahini-yogurt drizzle (p.85)
MID-AFTERNOON SNACK:	▶ Handful of strawberries
DINNER:	▶ Blinis with roasted spiced cauliflower (p.105)

DAY 1: MINDFULNESS PLAN

SOAK IT UP

'You time' is important. Today, make a point of having some! Take a long bath with delicious scents and soft bubbles. Luxuriate in this extended, peaceful moment.

DAY 1: BODYWEIGHT RESISTANCE

1 REVERSE LUNGE WITH FRONT KICK

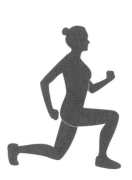

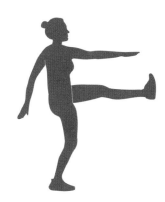

1 Stand tall, feet hip-width apart, relax your shoulders and look straight ahead. Engage your abs by pulling your navel in towards your spine.

2 Take a large step back with your left foot, planting your foot, toes downwards and tucked under. Lower your body until both legs are bent in right-angles. Lean forwards slightly to increase the work for your glutes and hamstrings.

3 Exhale, straighten your legs and lift your left foot off the floor behind you, bringing your knee forwards, still in the right-angle position, so that your left knee comes towards your chest. Don't stop here! Keep going and launch an explosive front kick with your left leg. Come back to starting position, and then in a continuous motion step back with your right foot, repeating the kick on the right side. Repeat with alternating legs for 1 minute.

2 SQUAT WITH WOOD CHOP

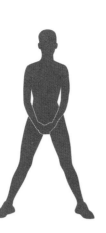
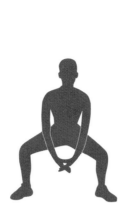

1 Stand tall, feet shoulder-width apart and pointing forwards. Relax your shoulders and look straight ahead. Interlink your fingers in front of you (you can hold a weight or dumbbell in both hands if you like), arms hanging down.

2 Bending at your knees, dig your heels into the floor and lower, back straight, abs engaged and lower back neutral. Push your hips backwards until your thighs are parallel to the floor. Don't extend your knees beyond your toes; keep your hands together. Arms bent at the elbows, twist left, moving your hands to the outside of your left leg.

3 Exhale, and turn right again, at the same time pushing up with your legs, lifting your hands diagonally across your body, rotating from your torso, to fully extend to the right, arms above your head. Pivot on your left foot to extend your reach. Return to the starting position and repeat on the other side. Repeat the whole sequence for 1 minute.

3 GLUTE BRIDGE WITH ONE LEG EXTENDED

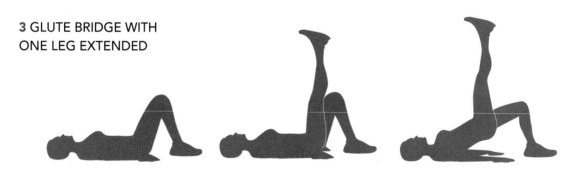

1 Lie on your back on the floor (use a mat for comfort), knees bent, feet flat on the floor, hip-width apart. Push your lower back into the floor to make sure your back isn't arched.

2 Extend your right leg straight upwards, with the sole of your foot towards the ceiling, and raise it off the floor, pushing down through your left foot to bring your bottom off the floor as you do so.

3 Extend the lift as far as you can, pause for 1–2 seconds, then lower, leg extended until it hovers just above the ground. Repeat the lift and lower on your right leg for 1 minute, then repeat on the left side.

4 GLUTE KICKBACK (2)

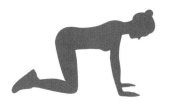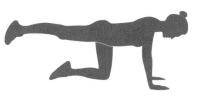

1 Start on the floor on all fours (use a mat for comfort). Position your hands roughly shoulder-width apart, directly under your shoulders, and ensure your knees are directly under your hips.

2 Engage your abs by pulling your navel towards your spine. Straighten your right leg and extended it behind you so that it's in line with your body and parallel to the floor.

3 Contract your glutes, and keeping your right leg straight, lift it up as high as possible. Then, with control, bring it down on a diagonal so that your right foot crosses your left ankle and touches down to the left your left foot. Repeat for 1 minute, then repeat using the left leg.

5 SINGLE LEG DEADLIFT

1 Stand tall, feet hip-width apart and well anchored. Transfer your weight to your right leg, ever-so-slightly bending your right knee (that is, not locked-out and totally straight). Raise your left foot a little off the ground. Engage your abs by pulling your navel towards your spine, and find your balance.

2 Pivot forwards at the hips, extending your left leg behind you. Keep your core engaged; avoid curving your back or hunching your shoulders. Slowly, with control lower your body and raise your left leg until it is parallel to the floor. Aim to create a T-shape with your legs and body. Allow your arms to hang down.

3 Slowly and with control, return to the starting position. Aim to dispatch 1 minute of continuous repetitions, extending and pivoting and returning to the start. Then, swap legs and repeat for a further 1 minute, standing on your left leg and extending your right leg behind you.

DAY 2

DAY 2: NUTRITION PLAN

BREAKFAST:	▶ Purple vitality (p.132), then Quinoa granola (p.55)
MID-MORNING SNACK:	▶ Energy balls (p.126)
LUNCH:	▶ Spiced lentil & artichoke salad (p.74)
MID-AFTERNOON SNACK:	▶ 1 apple
DINNER:	▶ Venison salad with fresh herb dressing (p.87)

DAY 2: MINDFULNESS PLAN

ENJOY THE PREPARATION

Did you know that digestion begins with the eyes? The time you spend preparing your food, looking at it and cooking it is time that your stomach is getting ready to receive it. Today, spend some extra time on the gathering, chopping, mixing and cooking – enjoy the sights and smells of making food, as well as of eating it!

DAY 2: LOW-INTENSITY POWER WALK

Remember this from Week 1? It's the day you secretly thought was a bit of a rest! Indeed, today should probably feel like a minor victory, because you're not tearing muscle fibres, dancing in the anaerobic zone-of-terror, or HIIT-ing your way up and down hills! It's another 1-hour power walk. Ideally, you'll get up nice and early, like last week, and get down to business and do the full hour. However, if you don't have a full 60 minutes to give first thing in the morning, aim for 30 minutes and then go for another 30 minutes in the evening. If it's practical, you could even get off your train or bus, or out of your car, 30 minutes from your workplace and power walk the rest of the way (and back again at the end of the day). Power walking is a super-convenient form of exercise – break it down and work it into your daily routine if you need to: a 10-minute brisk walk to fetch your morning cup of tea; a 20-minute post-lunch march around the city… However you do it, keep the pace up and power on!

DAY 3

DAY 3: NUTRITION PLAN

BREAKFAST:	▶ Energiser (p.132), then Eggs from the 'forest' (p.63)
MID-MORNING SNACK:	▶ Kale chips with za'atar (p.123)
LUNCH:	▶ Tuna, edamame & caper salad with mustard dressing (p.71)
MID-AFTERNOON SNACK:	▶ Handful of raspberries
DINNER:	▶ Marinated chicken with butternut squash & ginger mash (p.88)

DAY 3: MINDFULNESS PLAN

STRETCH

In this book, we've talked about the importance of stretching as a warm-up or cool-down for your body, but we also talked about how important it is to stretch just for the sake of stretching. Today, spend 10 minutes stretching out your body properly. Have a look at the stretches on pages 148–154 and stretch out your arms, legs, hips, back, neck and shoulders for your general wellbeing.

DAY 3: BODYWEIGHT RESISTANCE

1 BEAR CRAWLS

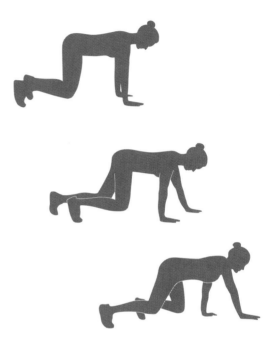

1 Start on the floor on all fours (use a mat for comfort), with your hands directly underneath your shoulders and your knees beneath your hips.

2 Push up onto your toes, raising your knees off the floor, but keeping them bent so that your back is completely straight and parallel to the ground (no arching or slouching). Engage your abs, by pulling your navel in towards your spine. Move forwards in a slow and controlled motion, starting with left arm and right leg forwards.

3 Then, switch to right arm, left leg, so that you're moving like a bear. At no point should your knees touch the floor, but roaring is optional. Move like this for 1 minute.

2 FULL PUSH-UP

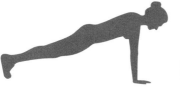 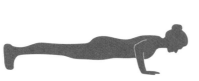 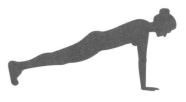

1 Lie face down on the floor. Place your hands to the sides and in line with your shoulders, in a wide grip. Tuck your toes under and push up on your arms so that you are in full plank position – spine straight, abdominals engaged, bottom in line with your back (take care not to sag or let your bottom lift too high).

2 When you're ready, inhale and lower yourself until your chest almost touches the floor. Keep your core strong (spine straight, abs engaged) and your body in a perfectly straight line.

3 Squeeze your chest, exhale and press your upper body back up to the starting position. Again, staying in perfect alignment throughout. After a brief pause at the top of the push-up, slowly and with control lower yourself again, repeating the full push-up as often as necessary for 1 minute.

3 FLYING SUPERMAN

1 Lie face down on the floor (use a mat for comfort). Extend your arms in front of your head and lengthen your legs behind you, soles of your feet pointing towards the ceiling. Let both legs rest on the floor.

2 Slowly and with control, as you exhale, simultaneously raise your arms, legs and chest off the floor. Squeeze your glutes to hold this super-demanding contraction for 2 seconds.

3 Inhale, and slowly and with control lower your arms, legs and chest to the floor, returning to your starting position. Repeat the raise and lower for 1 minute. It's kryptonite to many!

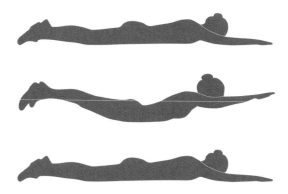

4 TRICEPS DIPS WITH KICKS

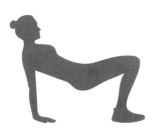 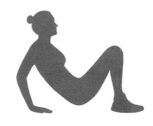 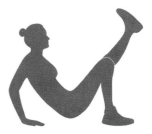

1 Sit upright on the floor with your back straight, knees bent with your feet flat on the floor and arms by your sides. Press your palms into the floor, straighten your arms and raise your bottom off the floor. Using your feet to anchor yourself, push as high as you can go without locking your elbows.

2 Keeping your elbows tucked in to your sides, slowly and with control bend your arms to lower your bottom and upper body towards the floor. Don't let your bottom touch the floor.

3 As you lower, raise your left leg up straight out in front and up so that your thighs are parallel and your left foot is flexed. Push down with your hands and use your triceps to lift yourself back to the starting position, simultaneously returning your left leg to the floor. Repeat, raising your right leg from the floor. Alternate legs for 1 minute.

5 SHOULDER PRESS PUSH UP

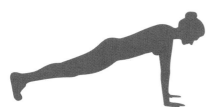 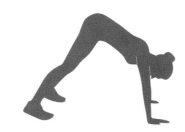 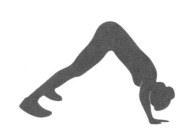

1 Start in a full plank position with your hands slightly wider than shoulder-width apart, abs engaged and body in perfect alignment. Take care not to let your bottom sag or come too high.

2 Push your hips towards the ceiling, rocking back on your toes, keeping your heels off the ground. At this point your body should be shaped like an upside-down 'V'.

3 Slowly and with control, lower your head towards the floor, bending your elbows as necessary. Just before your head touches the floor, pause, and then press back up to the starting position. Repeat the raise and lower, always staying in control, for 1 minute.

DAY 4

DAY 4: NUTRITION PLAN

BREAKFAST:	▶ Vitamin-C bomb (p.134); Apple & date mixed grain porridge (p.57)
MID-MORNING SNACK:	▶ Energy balls (p.126)
LUNCH:	▶ Scandi seaweed wraps (p.84)
MID-AFTERNOON SNACK:	▶ ¼ small watermelon
DINNER:	▶ Venison meatballs with blackberry sauce (p.90)

DAY 4: MINDFULNESS PLAN

HAVE A POINT-OF-FOCUS MASSAGE

Today, sit quietly and do a quick body-scan. Where can you feel any tightness? At this stage in the programme, your lower back and glutes could be feeling it in particular. Find a tennis ball and use it to massage out your tightest muscles. Lie on it and roll around on it to release tension in your back or glutes; hold it and roll it over sensitive areas on your shoulders; and so on. With appropriate pressure, it's an incredible release for your body – and mind!

DAY 4: HIIT PLAN

It's HIIT time again, and perhaps you've come to love it already?! We're going to mix it up a little this week, and keep it fresh. Today, find a local hill, or if you live on the Great Plains and a hill's not forthcoming, you can use a flight of stairs – either way, you'll need enough of a hill or enough stairs to make your activity burst at least 10 seconds long. Find a timer (likely on your phone), shoot up the hill, and then power walk (see p.159) down the hill in double the time. The walking down will effectively be your recovery period, and this will give you just enough time to lower your heart rate, steady your breathing, and return to more of a resting state to get to the bottom of the hill again, turn around and immediately shoot back up to the top again.

Aim to keep up the speed, with the same 1:2 ratio as last week's HIIT exercise: 10 seconds up the hill and then 20 seconds down it; or, if you really want to push it, 1 minute up the hill and then 2 minutes down it (or any combination in a 1:2 ratio). Aim for a total workout time of between 10 and 15 minutes.

DAY 5

DAY 5: NUTRITION PLAN

BREAKFAST:	▶ Wake-me-up (p.134), then Max muesli (p.56)
MID-MORNING SNACK:	▶ On-the-go power bar (p.125)
LUNCH:	▶ Rainbow salad with roasted spiced almonds (p.77)
MID-AFTERNOON SNACK:	▶ 1 peach
DINNER:	▶ Swedish crayfish party (p.100)

DAY 5: MINDFULNESS PLAN

KEEP TRACK

Find a notebook and pen, or use the note function on your smartphone, and keep a record of everything you eat today and at what time. Capture your emotional reflections on your daily routine. This time next week, revisit your annotations to see how your views are developing.

DAY 5: BODYWEIGHT RESISTANCE

1 WALKING PLANK WITH SIDE PLANK

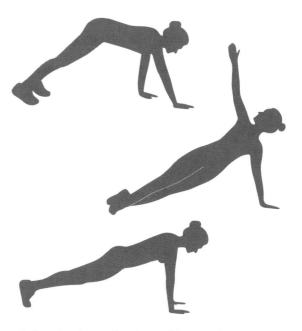

1 Stand with your feet hip-width apart. Engage your abs and bend forwards from your hips to plant your right and then left hands on the floor in front of you. Walk your hands forwards, raising your heels until you reach full plank position with your body in complete alignment from head to toe.

2 Push your weight into your left hand and lift your right hand off the floor, turning your whole body at the same time, but keeping its alignment.

3 Hold the side plank for 3–5 seconds, then carefully return to the full plank position (as shown) and repeat on the other side, this time raising your left hand. Return to full plank, then walk your hands back until you have returned to standing. Repeat steps 1–3 for 1 minute.

2 SINGLE LEG BURPEES

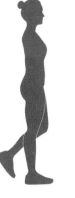

1 Stand straight with your feet hip-width apart and arms by your sides. Lift your left leg off the floor, hovering your left toes above the ground.

2 Drop your hands to the floor, planting them slightly wider than shoulder-width apart, keeping your left toes off the ground the whole time.

3 Jump back with your right leg, extending your raised left leg. Keep your abs engaged and jump your right foot back towards your hands, drop your left foot to the floor and return to starting position. Switch legs and repeat. Keep alternating for 1 minute.

---

3 MOUNTAIN CLIMBER

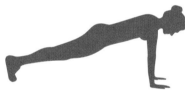 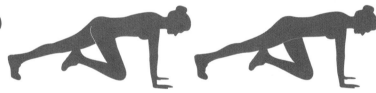

1 Begin by putting yourself into a full press-up position – feet hip-width apart, toes tucked under, raised up on your straightened (but not locked) elbows, spine in perfect alignment and shoulders over your wrists. Engage your abs by pulling your navel in towards your spine.

2 Bring your right knee forwards towards your right arm and touch the tops of your right toes to the floor. In a continuous 'running' movement, return your right leg back to the starting position.

3 As you do so, bring your left knee forwards towards your left arm, touching the tops of your left toes to the ground. How far forwards you can touch will depend on your flexibility. Go as far as you can, maintaining a straight spine throughout (don't raise your bottom). Keep the tempo high, alternating legs in and out as if two pistons are firing alternately. Continue for 1 minute, or until you have to stop.

4 FULL TURKISH GET-UPS

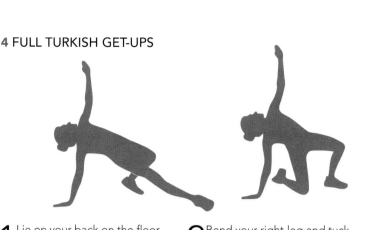

1 Lie on your back on the floor (use a mat for comfort), with your legs straight out in front of you and your arms by your sides. Follow the beginner sequence on page 185, then from the almost-seated position, drive your weight through your left heel to bring yourself into a sort of side plank.

2 Bend your right leg and tuck it behind your left heel, toes under. Your weight is on your left foot and right arm. Pivot your left leg at the knee, sweeping your left foot to towards your left hand, straightening your body to face forwards, but still looking at your left hand.

3 Push into your left foot and use your left thigh to bring yourself to standing (keeping your left arm raised throughout). Unwind the movement, reversing each step so that you return to lying on your back. Repeat for 1 minute on this side, then for 1 minute on the other side.

5 BICYCLE KICKS

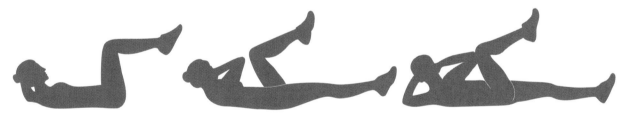

1 Sit on your bottom on the floor, legs out in front of you (use a mat for comfort), arms bent at the elbows and hands on either side of your head. Lean back, keeping your head raised, engage your abdominals and raise your legs off the floor, bending them at the knees and so that your thighs are perpendicular to the floor. Keep your ankles soft.

2 From the hip, bring your left knee towards your chest. Your right leg should extend but remain off the floor. At the same time, reach your right elbow to touch your left knee as it comes towards your chest. Take care not to pull on your head – just rest your fingers on the sides of your head and use your abdominals to create the reach.

3 Return to the starting position and immediately bring your right knee up to your chest and reach towards it with your left elbow. Return to the starting position. Continue to alternate left knee to right elbow and right knee to left elbow, keeping your legs raised from the floor, for 1 minute. Try to keep a good pace throughout.

DAY 6

DAY 6: NUTRITION PLAN

BREAKFAST:	▶ Energiser (p.132), then Baked avocado with egg & trout tartare (p.60)
MID-MORNING SNACK:	▶ Kale chips with za'atar (p.123)
LUNCH:	▶ Simple salad with crayfish & citrus dressing (p.72)
MID-AFTERNOON SNACK:	▶ handful of blueberries
DINNER:	▶ Venison salad with fresh herb dressing (p.87)

DAY 6: MINDFULNESS PLAN

CUT THE CANDY-FLOSS

Psychological 'empty calories' or media 'junk food' is as unhealthy for the brain as fast food is for the body! They can sap countless hours and most of your energy, leaving you feeling emotionally and mentally empty. Today, avoid tumbling down the Insta-rabbit hole, flicking through the infinite reel of social media and entering online-video vortices and see how much more of real benefit you can achieve!

DAY 6 AND 7: REST DAYS

Days 6 and 7 are your rest days – remember how relieved you were when you got to this bit in Week 1? As before, though, stretching out your body is always good for you. So, if you feel like it, wake up on these days and practise your Sun Salutation (see pp.28–32 for full explanation) and in the process give your body a good stretch out for the day ahead. Begin in Mountain Pose, and then follow the sequence shown on the right, reversing it once you get to the end.

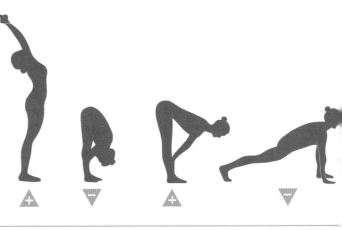

DAY 7

DAY 7: NUTRITION PLAN

BREAKFAST:	▶ Purple vitality (p.132), then Sundae for Sunday (p.58)
MID-MORNING SNACK:	▶ Roasted spiced almonds (p.122)
LUNCH:	▶ Marinated salmon with fennel (p.82)
MID-AFTERNOON SNACK:	▶ 1 red pepper, sliced
DINNER:	▶ Poached eggs on smoky garlic chickpeas with smashed broad beans (p.104)

DAY 7: MINDFULNESS PLAN

HIGHLIGHT THE POSITIVES

Note down three positive things that you've accomplished with your health in the recent past. It could be anything that is personal and true to you: 'I've walked more this week than I normally do', 'I've eaten and prepared more fresh foods', 'I'm feeling stronger and lifting heavier.' It's all too easy to focus on the things we don't achieve, beating ourselves up for our apparent failings, and we forget that it's also important to give ourselves a pat on the back to recognise the good work we're putting in.

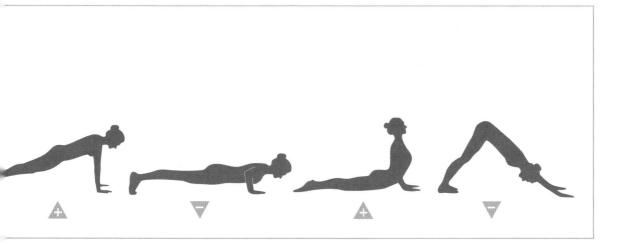

WEEK 3

'Fit is not a destination, it's a way of life.'

ANONYMOUS

It's said to take three weeks to form a habit. In embarking on your third week, you've now firmly committed to yourself. Hopefully, your commitment is becoming a routine, and that routine is becoming easier. You'll likely notice some exercises becoming less strenuous already. Stick to your guns; the next step is to carry on, to keep training, and to keep augmenting your routine with incrementally higher repetitions, shorter recovery periods and stronger resolve! Great work so far, now let's smash this final week!

DAY 1

DAY 1: NUTRITION PLAN

BREAKFAST:	▶ Wake-me-up (p.134), then Quinoa granola (p.55)
MID-MORNING SNACK:	▶ Roasted spiced almonds (see p.122)
LUNCH:	▶ Spiced lentil & artichoke salad (p.74)
MID-AFTERNOON SNACK:	▶ ½ cucumber, cut into sticks
DINNER:	▶ Blinis with roasted spiced cauliflower (p.105)

DAY 1: MINDFULNESS PLAN

TRAVEL AS WELL AS ARRIVE

Your mind and your body need water. As clichéd as it may sound, in a world that is so results-orientated, take some time to enjoy the journey. Stop what you're doing and think about enjoying the healthier eating, the deeper, stronger training, and even the soreness on the following days! Savour it all.

DAY 1: BODYWEIGHT RESISTANCE

1 JUMPING LUNGES

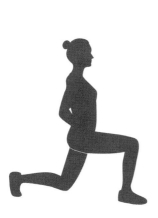
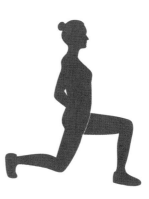

1 Stand tall, feet hip-width apart, relax your shoulders and look straight ahead. Engage your core by pulling your navel towards your spine, tuck your hands behind your back. Take a large step back with your left foot, tucking your toes under. Lower until both legs are at right-angles. Lean forwards slightly to increase the work for your glutes and hamstrings.

2 Pause, then push off with a springing jump, going as high as you possibly can, and keeping your hands behind your back. Look forwards.

3 Switch your legs around in mid-air so that when you land your right foot is at the back and your left foot is in front. Repeat the lift-off, switching legs each time, for 1 minute.

2 STATIC SQUAT WITH JUMP

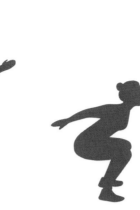

1 Stand tall and plant your feet shoulder-width apart, relax your shoulders and look straight ahead. Point your feet forwards, bend your arms at the elbows, so that your fingers point forwards, too.

2 Bending at your knees and digging your heels into the floor, push your hips backwards to lower yourself until your legs are parallel with the floor. Keep your back straight, your abs engaged and your lower back as neutral as possible. Avoid allowing your knees to extend beyond your toes. Swing your arms back.

3 Press down into the floor and explosively jump up into the air, landing with soft knees in the starting position. Repeat the sequence of squat then jump continuously for 1 minute.

3 GLUTE BRIDGE WITH ONE LEG EXTENDED

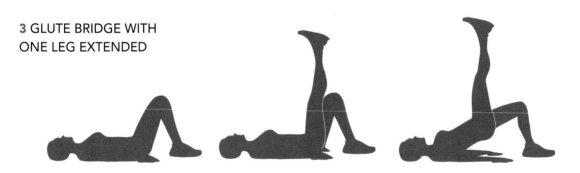

1 Lie on your back on the floor (use a mat for comfort), knees bent, feet flat on the floor, hip-width apart. Push your lower back into the floor to make sure your back isn't arched.

2 Extend your right leg straight upwards, with the sole of your foot towards the ceiling, and raise it off the floor, pushing down through your left foot to bring your bottom off the floor as you do so.

3 Extend the lift as far as you can, pause for 1–2 seconds, then lower, leg extended until it hovers just above the ground. Repeat the lift and lower on your right leg for 1 minute, then repeat on the left side.

4 GLUTE KICKBACK (3)

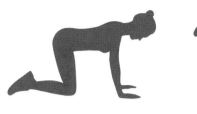
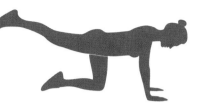

1 Start on the floor on all fours (use a mat for comfort). Position your hands roughly shoulder-width apart, directly under your shoulders, and ensure your knees are directly under your hips.

2 Pull your navel towards your spine to engage your abs. Straighten your right leg and extended it behind you so that it's in line with your body and parallel to the floor. Contract your glutes and, keeping your right leg straight, lift it as high as possible.

3 Keeping your leg raised as high and as straight as possible, move your right foot in circular wand-like motions for 1 minute. Lower your right leg to the floor, then repeat the sequence with your left leg raised for a further 1 minute.

---

5 SINGLE LEG DEADLIFT

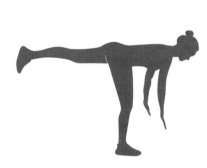

1 Stand tall, feet hip-width apart and well anchored. Transfer your weight to your right leg, ever-so-slightly bending your right knee (that is, not locked-out and totally straight). Raise your left foot a little off the ground. Engage your abs by pulling your navel towards your spine, and find your balance.

2 Pivot forwards at the hips, extending your left leg behind you. Keep your core engaged; avoid curving your back or hunching your shoulders. Slowly, with control lower your body and raise your left leg until it is parallel to the floor. Aim to create a T-shape with your legs and body. Allow your arms to hang down.

3 Slowly and with control, return to the starting position. Aim to dispatch 1 minute of continuous repetitions, extending and pivoting and returning to the start. Then, swap legs and repeat for a further 1 minute, standing on your left leg and extending your right leg behind you.

DAY 2

DAY 2: NUTRITION PLAN

BREAKFAST:	▶ Rocket fuel (p.131), then Tofu & spring onion pancakes (p.61)
MID-MORNING SNACK:	▶ On-the-go power bar (p.125)
LUNCH:	▶ Tuna, edamame & caper salad with mustard dressing (p.71)
MID-AFTERNOON SNACK:	▶ 1 banana
DINNER:	▶ Marinated chicken with butternut squash & ginger mash (p.88)

DAY 2: LOW-INTENSITY POWER WALK

It hardly feels appropriate to say 'final push now', seeing as power walking isn't about the last burst for the finish line. It's slow, steady, and achievably relentless in its pace. Today, your power walking day of Week 3, it might feel as though you've started to form a habit: you'll have set the alarm a little earlier, thrown on your trainers, and looked forwards to hitting the pavement for 60 minutes of walking the beat! As you go, try to remember how great it feels to be outdoors, to appreciate the beauty around you. If it's grey, drizzling and dark, I hear you; that's pretty hard – at that point you just have to grit your teeth and power through. But if it's a half-decent day, that should be all the inspiration you need to get out there – breathe deep and walk hard!

DAY 2: MINDFULNESS PLAN

REBOOT WITH NATURE

Spending time outdoors has been proven to yield feelings of calm, as well as providing a natural energy boost. Today, whether it's part of your fitness routine or simply a quiet moment on your terrace or patio or in your local park, spend some time outdoors, drinking in all the sights, smells and sounds of nature.

DAY 3

DAY 3: NUTRITION PLAN

BREAKFAST:	▶ Energiser (p.132), then Quinoa granola (p.55)
MID-MORNING SNACK:	▶ Kale chips with za'atar (p.123)
LUNCH:	▶ Broad bean, mint & ricotta smörgås (p.78)
MID-AFTERNOON SNACK:	▶ 1 grapefruit
DINNER:	▶ Prawn, anchovy & greens pasta (p.99)

DAY 3: MINDFULNESS PLAN

WALK TO THINK

Take some time for a gentle walk in your local park or, as we love to in Sweden, in the forest if you have one nearby. Walking has been said to focus the mind and allow the right space and pace for some introspection and reflection. I do some of my best thinking when alone, just walking.

DAY 3: BODYWEIGHT RESISTANCE

1 BEAR CRAWLS

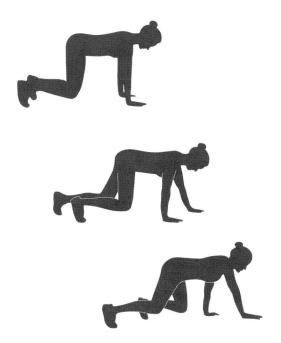

1 Start on the floor on all fours (use a mat for comfort), with your hands directly underneath your shoulders and your knees beneath your hips.

2 Push up onto your toes, raising your knees off the floor, but keeping them bent so that your back is completely straight and parallel to the ground (no arching or slouching). Engage your abs, by pulling your navel in towards your spine. Move forwards in a slow and controlled motion, starting with left arm and right leg forwards.

3 Then, switch to right arm, left leg, so that you're moving like a bear. At no point should your knees touch the floor, but roaring is optional. Move like this for 1 minute.

2 NARROW GRIP PUSH-UP

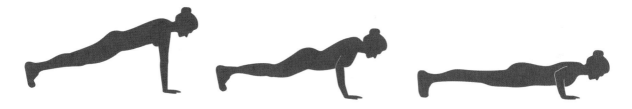

1 Lie face down on the floor. Place your hands in line with your shoulders, elbows tight against your sides, which will work your triceps hard. Tuck your toes under and push up on your arms so that you are in a perfect plank – spine straight, abs engaged, bottom in line (take care not to sag or let it lift too high).

2 When you're ready, inhale and start to lower yourself towards the floor. Keep your core strong (spine straight, abs engaged) and your body in a perfectly straight line. The movement is slow and with control.

3 Keep lowering until your chest almost touches the floor. Then. squeeze your chest, exhale and press your upper body back up to the starting position, staying in perfect alignment throughout. After a brief pause at the top, lower yourself again, repeating the full push-up as often as necessary for 1 minute.

3 KNEELING SUPERMAN

1 This is a multiplex exercise! It's more demanding than other supermen, because balance and core engagement are thrown together. Start by kneeling on all fours. Position your hands roughly shoulder-width apart, directly beneath your shoulders, and ensure your knees are directly beneath your hips. Cushion your knees with a folded towel for comfort, if you like.

2 Engage your abdominals and extend your left leg out behind your body as far as you can, kneeling on your right leg for support. Care not to tilt your hips, keeping them square to the floor. At the same time, extend your right arm outwards in front of your body as far as you can.

3 Return your arm and leg back to your torso, but not to the floor. Instead, extend again in a slow and controlled manner. Repeat this movement for 1 minute. (There's no better way to train for saving Lois Lane!) After the first minute, return to starting position and repeat the sequence using your right leg and left arm for a further 1 minute.

4 TRICEPS DIPS WITH KICKS

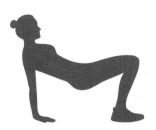 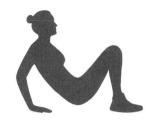 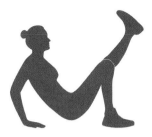

1 Sit upright on the floor with your back straight, knees bent with your feet flat on the floor and arms by your sides. Press your palms into the floor, straighten your arms and raise your bottom off the floor. Using your feet to anchor yourself, push as high as you can go without locking your elbows.

2 Keeping your elbows tucked in to your sides, slowly and with control bend your arms to lower your bottom and upper body towards the floor. Don't let your bottom touch the floor.

3 As you lower, raise your left leg up straight out in front and up so that your thighs are parallel and your left foot is flexed. Push down with your hands and use your triceps to lift yourself back to the starting position, simultaneously returning your left leg to the floor. Repeat, raising your right leg from the floor. Alternate legs for 1 minute.

5 UPPER BACK BLASTER

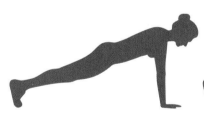 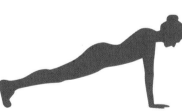 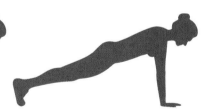

1 Lie face down on a mat on the floor, tuck your toes under and raise yourself onto your hands to put yourself into a plank position. Ensure you have a straight spine and you fire up your abdominals by drawing your navel in towards your spine. Relax your shoulders and neck muscles such that they're not bunched up towards your ears. You need a soft and neutral posture.

2 Slowly squeeze your shoulder blades together as hard and as much as you can without pain. Imagine you're squeezing something long and thin, like a stick, between your shoulder blades and trying to hold it there. Hold for 2–3 seconds, keeping your core strong and your body aligned throughout.

3 Release and return to your starting position, softening the posture once more. Repeat the squeeze, hold and release sequence for 1 minute. (Note: if you find this hard to do in the full plank, you can try it supporting yourself on your elbows, rather than your hands, in a low plank position.)

DAY 4

DAY 4: NUTRITION PLAN

BREAKFAST:	▶ Wake-me-up (p.134), then Apple & date mixed grain porridge (p.57)
MID-MORNING SNACK:	▶ Energy balls (p.126)
LUNCH:	▶ Asian broth with chicken & mint (p.67)
MID-AFTERNOON SNACK:	▶ 1 glass of (real) coconut water
DINNER:	▶ Venison meatballs with blackberry sauce (p.90)

DAY 4: MINDFULNESS PLAN

STEER YOUR THOUGHTS

By listening to your internal monologue, especially regarding your fitness, you might pick up on repeated negative thoughts: 'I can't do this', or perhaps 'I have too far to go.' Flip your thoughts on their heads. Instead, tell yourself, with your real voice, that you can do it, that you're nearly there, that you'll keep going. If you dream it, believe it and work for it, you're one step closer. Don't let your thoughts control or undermine you.

DAY 4: HIIT PLAN

This is it! Your final HIIT session (don't cheer too loudly!), and it's critical to keep changing it up so that you don't get 'workout fatigue', as that just kills motivation. Today, grab a skipping rope, set the stopwatch on your mobile phone and press GO! Stand up tall, and look up to keep a good posture and good balance. Slide your shoulder blades down away from you ears. Start skipping (the jumping kind rather than the running kind). Land on the balls of your feet and be nimble. I recommend that you try not to jump metres up into the air, Michael Jordan-style. A few centimetres is all you need to clear the rope and maintain minimum joint impact at the same time. Plus, you'll find small jumps easier to sustain for a longer period.

I find that a solid minute of fast-paced skipping can be super-challenging, so I'd suggest small increments for this HIIT session. Aim for 30 seconds of fast skipping followed by 1 minute of slow, recovery skipping, and repeat for 12 minutes in total. That should do the trick nicely, and allow you to complete eight cycles of HIIT skipping drills! If you're feeling super-bold, or finding it too easy (in which case well done, you're a champ!), try quickening the pace, or (better) adding 'high knees' for 1 minute followed by a more relaxed slow skip for 2 minutes, making your workout 15 minutes altogether.

DAY 5

DAY 5: NUTRITION PLAN

BREAKFAST:	▶ Purple vitality (p.132), then Max muesli (p.56)
MID-MORNING SNACK:	▶ Savoury egg muffin (p.128)
LUNCH:	▶ Scandi seaweed wraps (p.84)
MID-AFTERNOON SNACK:	▶ 1 pomegranate
DINNER:	▶ Warm salad of roasted salmon, fennel & baby new potatoes (p.93)

DAY 5: MINDFULNESS PLAN

MIRROR, MIRROR, ON THE WALL

If you're feeling a little mediocre, a tried-and-tested strategy is to go somewhere private with a full-length mirror, and get yourself pumped up, as a boxer might do before a fight. Flex your muscles, dance like a butterfly, sting like a bee, gee yourself up... and then head out to the real world. You'll tackle it with WAY more energy!

DAY 5: UPPER BODY PLAN

1 WALKING PLANK WITH SIDE PLANK

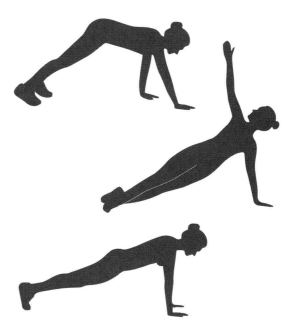

1 Stand with your feet hip-width apart. Engage your abs and bend forwards from your hips to plant your right and then left hands on the floor in front of you. Walk your hands forwards, raising your heels until you reach full plank position with your body in complete alignment from head to toe.

2 Push your weight into your left hand and lift your right hand off the floor, turning your whole body at the same time, but keeping its alignment.

3 Hold the side plank for 3–5 seconds, then carefully return to the full plank position (as shown) and repeat on the other side, this time raising your left hand. Return to full plank, then walk your hands back until you have returned to standing. Repeat steps 1–3 for 1 minute.

2 SINGLE LEG BURPEES

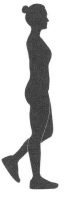
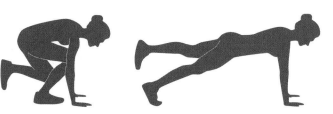

1 Stand straight with your feet hip-width apart and arms by your sides. Lift your left leg off the floor, hovering your left toes above the ground.

2 Drop your hands to the floor, planting them slightly wider than shoulder-width apart, keeping your left toes off the ground the whole time.

3 Jump back with your right leg, extending your raised left leg. Keep your abs engaged and jump your right foot back towards your hands, drop your left foot to the floor and return to starting position. Swtich legs and repeat. Keep alternating for 1 minute.

---

3 MOUNTAIN CLIMBER

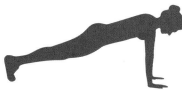
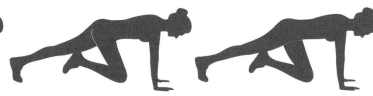

1 Begin by putting yourself into a full press-up position – feet hip-width apart, toes tucked under, raised up on your straightened (but not locked) elbows, spine in perfect alignment and shoulders over your wrists. Engage your abs by pulling your navel in towards your spine.

2 Bring your right knee forwards towards your right arm and touch the tops of your right toes to the floor. In a continuous 'running' movement, return your right leg back to the starting position.

3 As you do so, bring your left knee forwards towards your left arm, touching the tops of your left toes to the ground. How far forwards you can touch will depend on your flexibility. Go as far as you can, maintaining a straight spine throughout (don't raise your bottom). Keep the tempo high, alternating legs in and out as if two pistons are firing alternately. Continue for 1 minute, or until you have to stop.

4 FULL TURKISH GET-UPS

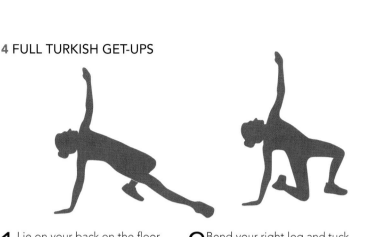

1 Lie on your back on the floor (use a mat for comfort), with your legs straight out in front of you and your arms by your sides. Follow the beginner sequence on page 185, then from the almost-seated position, drive your weight through your left heel to bring yourself into a sort of side plank.

2 Bend your right leg and tuck it behind your left heel, toes under. Your weight is on your left foot and right arm. Pivot your left leg at the knee, sweeping your left foot to towards your left hand, straightening your body to face forwards, but still looking at your left hand.

3 Push into your left foot and use your left thigh to bring yourself to standing (keeping your left arm raised throughout). Unwind the movement, reversing each step so that you return to lying on your back. Repeat for 1 minute on this side, then for 1 minute on the other side.

5 REVERSE CRUNCH

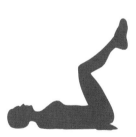 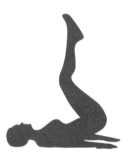 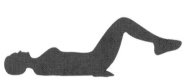

1 Lie on your back on the floor (use a mat for comfort), taking care not to arch your back, arms by your sides, palms down. Place your feet together flat on the floor so that your legs are slightly bent at the knee, then hinge at your hips to raise your feet off the floor until your toes point upwards.

2 Keeping your feet together use your abs to bring your legs towards your chest, so that your thighs are perpendicular to the floor (or a little further if you can) and your hips and bottom lift off the floor. Hold this position for 1–2 seconds.

3 Use your abs to mastermind the movement as you lower your feet back towards the floor, slowly and with control. Repeat the reverse crunch as often as you can for 1 minute.

DAY 6

DAY 6: NUTRITION PLAN

BREAKFAST:	▶ Immune booster (p.135), Baked avocado with egg & trout tartare (p.60)
MID-MORNING SNACK:	▶ Three-nut butter (p.124) with fruit or on toast
LUNCH:	▶ Mini chickpea burgers with tahini-yogurt drizzle (p.85)
MID-AFTERNOON SNACK:	▶ 1 apple
DINNER:	▶ Seafood & fennel tagine with saffron aioli (p.96)

DAY 6: MINDFULNESS PLAN

... AND BREATHE

It's all too easy to hold your stomach tense with stress the whole day. Take a few minutes today to focus on breathing deeply. Aim for whole belly-filling breaths, at a steady pace. Breathe in through your nose right down deep into your abdomen (don't stop at your chest!) and slowly out through your mouth. Feel the tension ebb away.

DAY 6 AND 7: REST DAYS

We're here again! Days 6 and 7 are your rest days – you've come so far, surely you are ready for a rest? Same rules apply, though – stretching is good for you! So, if you feel like it, wake up on these days and practise your Salute to the Sun (see pp.28–32 for full explanation) and in the process give your body a good stretch out for the day ahead. Begin in Mountain Pose, and then follow the sequence shown on the right, reversing it once you get to the end.

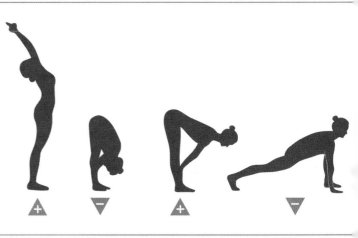

DAY 7

DAY 7: NUTRITION PLAN

BREAKFAST:	▶ Super-vit (p.131), then Sundae for Sunday (p.58)
MID-MORNING SNACK:	▶ Roasted spiced almonds (see p.122)
LUNCH:	▶ Marinated salmon with fennel (p.82)
MID-AFTERNOON SNACK:	▶ Handful of blueberries
DINNER:	▶ Wild mushroom & spelt risotto (p.103)

DAY 7: MINDFULNESS PLAN

CELEBRATE!

You did it! Today is the last day of the three-week plan and you made it here. Not anyone else – just you. Today, hold yourself tall and feel proud. You're a champ!

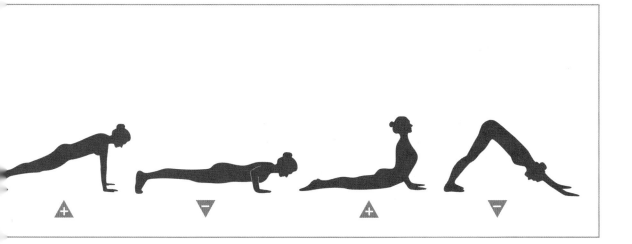

BEYOND WEEK THREE

By now you've completed your three-week plan and should be well on your way to arming yourself with the right tools to stay Scandi-fit year-in, year-out. Following your three weeks of rebooting, you're now more ready than ever to adopt a permanently healthy mindset and lifestyle. You have everything you need, now it's up to you!

DON'T GIVE UP

Remember, you are creating a new, healthier lifestyle, and what matters most is that you don't give up. Throwing in the towel is the only thing that guarantees you won't get the results you want. Precision is everything, quality over quantity. Continue focusing on your form to ensure you get the most out of your workouts and you feel you're making progress. And remember that poor technique can be dangerous and ineffective, as well as dangerously ineffective! Stay focused, stay safe and never give up!

STAY ON THE PATH

The ideal future is one in which you prioritise and schedule your training so that it simply becomes consumed within your daily life – much like a business meeting you won't have an excuse to cancel. However, if you ever miss a meal or a training session, don't beat yourself up. Accept it and move on. Falling off the wagon is not a problem: it's inevitable, it's human, and you haven't 'failed'. Enjoy your treat (in whatever form it comes – a missed HIIT day, an indulgent chocolate pudding, a boozy night out with friends), and then get back on the wagon so that you haven't wasted your fall. It would be far worse to think 'Oh, I ate an extra cake, so I may as well embark upon a multi-day binge.' Accept the additional cake, enjoy it and move on. The same goes with training – if you miss one session, don't think 'I'll start over on Monday' and let the rest of the week go, too. Accept that you missed one session and get straight back to your training schedule tomorrow. Life is always going to throw things at you that might send you off-track. The best you can do is to go with it but to keep your structure ready to guide you back as soon as possible. The world isn't a stop–start plan; you just keep on going.

CHALLENGE YOUR BODY

Carry on changing up your workouts: introduce new exercises, add more resistance and keep it varied to make the whole thing fun and motivating. 'The same' will leave you like Bill Murray in *Groundhog Day*; 'different' will keep it fresh and challenging! YouTube is a wonderful resource for inspiration on how to mix it up. Perhaps in a month, go back to some of the earlier sections and chapters, sniff around them a little online, elaborate upon them further. Or, partner up with a friend and have a little training session together at the park once a week, making use of the three-week training plan as a guide to what you might like to do.

TINGLE YOUR TASTE BUDS

Keep raiding and tucking into the recipe section, too. Explore the wealth of recipe know-how online to use the ingredients in different ways – with different spices, textures and accompaniments. When you're at the supermarket, think about how to read the food labels and really digest what they're telling you; keep in mind what's a healthy amount of fat, what's the right type of sugar and so on.

FOCUS YOUR MIND

If you've had a tough day at work, recall your learnings around mindfulness. Treat yourself to a 5-minute break for a quick doodle, or maybe even a meditation mini-break. Search around on the Internet for more practical applications of mindfulness and adopt them into your daily life. If you've loved the idea of giving yourself a few minutes at the start of the day to collect your thoughts, consider turning it into more formal meditation 'me-time'. Keep searching and learning and extending your practice in ways that benefit your mind and your body.

My hope is that altogether, this three-week window into a Scandinavian-flavoured life – congratulations! You did it! – has inspired you to want to try new, healthier ways of living, and may have shown you that healthy can be easy, long-lasting and fun!

Lycka till (good luck)!

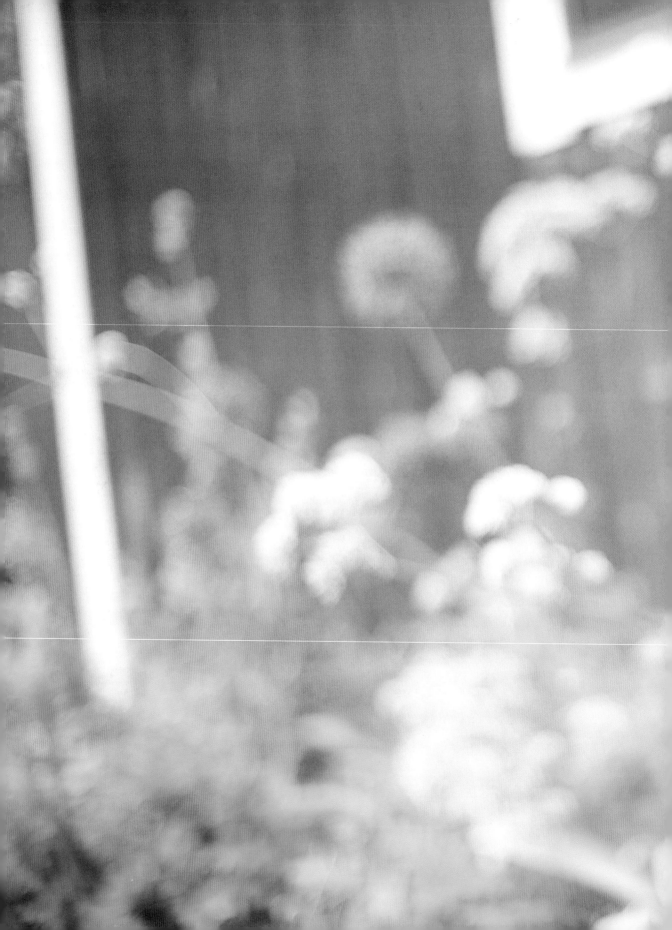

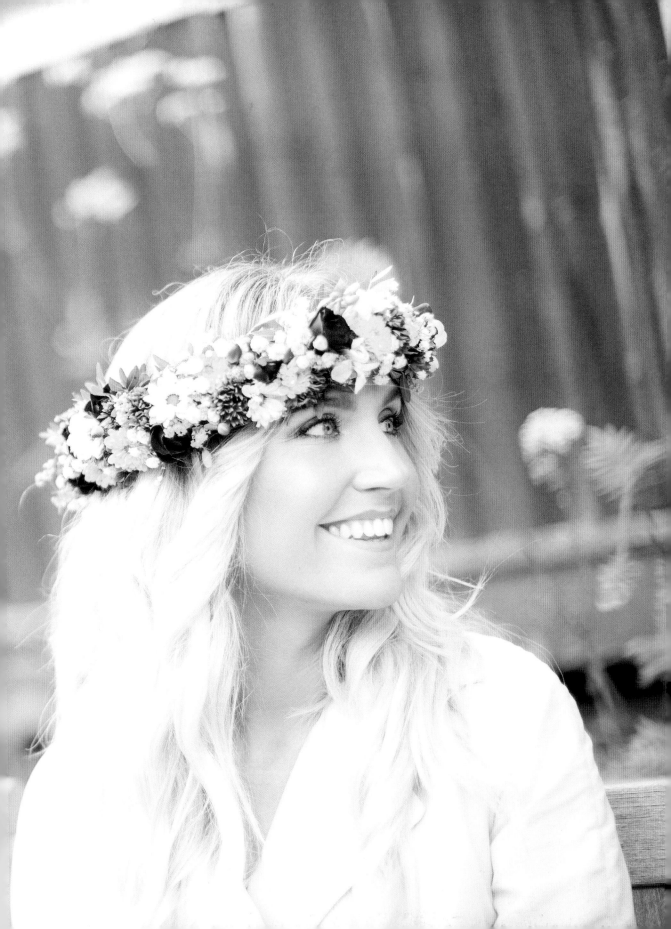

GENERAL INDEX

RECIPE INDEX

ACKNOWLEDGEMENTS

Firstly, without those who've subscribed to my blog and social media pages, this twisting and turning literary journey of mine would never have happened, so my untold thanks to you for following my escapades so far – I hope we share many more healthy shenanigans in the future. Also, thank you Oli for your professionalism, drive and dedication (and of course for your beautiful photography); Dad for your endless positivity, generous spirit, and giving me the confidence to be myself; Linnea for your friendship and loyalty; and Nicholas for always being 'on it' with such superb commitment! Finally, huge thank you to Hannah for believing there was a book in me – it's been an honour working with you.

Huge thanks also to the following companies for their continued support, helping me to create and grow alongside them!
• adidas (www.adidas.co.uk) • Helly Hansen (www.hellyhansen.com) • Monreal London (www.monreallondon.com)

Faya x